Contents

Part III   Conclusions

Contributors

Peter J. Franks
Director of Research, Centre for Research and Implementation of Clinical Practice at Thames Valley University

Suzanne Kite
Senior Registrar in Palliative Medicine, The Margaret Centre, Whiggs Cross Hospital, London

Maria Lorentzon
Research Fellow, Department of Primary Health Care and General Practice, Imperial College School of Medicine, London

Anne Naysmith
Palliative Care Consultant, Parkside Health Hospital, Pembridge Palliative Care Centre, St Charles Hospital, London

Emma K. Wilkinson
Project Researcher, Department of Primary Health Care and General Practice, Imperial College School of Medicine, London

Acknowledgements

Our late colleague, Debra Weston, worked on this project until her tragic death in an accident in August 1996. We appreciate the work she did and it reminds us of the loss for us all.

We would like to acknowledge the work of Matthew Wilkinson in designing the Access database and also for his advice on data entry. We also thank Alison Lee for her work in locating and photocopying articles, and Selina Salisbury for entering the data.

We would also like to acknowledge the assistance of the librarians at Imperial College School of Medicine for their help in devising and carrying out the online searches. We also thank the librarians at the Halley Stewart Library at St Christopher's Hospice and the British Medical Association library for their help in retrieving obscure articles.

We would also like to acknowledge all those researchers who responded to our request for information. The following individuals and organizations kindly sent us reference lists, unpublished papers, or other information:

- **Organizations**: Association for Palliative Medicine, Association for Palliative Medicine of Great Britain and Ireland, British Medical Association, Cochrane Collaboration, Department of Health, Earl Mountbatten Hospice, Galway Hospice Service, Institute of Cancer Research, Marie Curie Cancer Centre, Medical Research Council, Royal College of General Practitioners, St Christopher's Hospice, Trent Palliative Care Centre, United Kingdom Children's Cancer Study Group, Wellcome Trust.

- **Individuals**: Gerda Gibbs, Ian Johnson, Nik Cawley, Sue Duke, Dr Julia Addington Hall, Dr David Clark, Professor Jessica Corner, Professor Ilora Finlay, Dr Gillian Ford, Professor Irene Higginson, Ian Johnson, Dr Hugh Markowe, Dr Mark McCarthy, Mary Mullins, Dr Bill Noble, Marilyn Relf, Margaret Rogers, Dr Margaret Robbins, Dr Dave Seamark, Dr Neil Small, Dr Adrian Tookman, Susan Volker, Hellen Woolley.

A shortened version of 'Question 7: Impact on quality of life' has previously been published in the Journal 'Palliative Medicine'

(Salisbury, C., Bosanquet, N., Wilkinson, E., Franks, P.J., Kite, S., Lorentzon, M., and Naysmith, A. The impact of different models of specialist palliative care on patients' quality of life: A systematic literature review). Copyright material is reproduced here by kind permission of the editor.

Finally, we would like to acknowledge the support of the NHS Executive, which funded the project.

I

Introduction and methodology

1

Summary

Aims

The aim of this review was to identify the most appropriate and cost-effective models of service delivery and level of provision of palliative care services. This included the role of nurse practitioners in hospitals and the community, and the care of patients dying in acute hospitals.

Objectives

Within this aim 10 key research questions were identified, including the current need for and provision of services, proposed alternative models of provision, appropriate skill mix in nursing, the relationship between alternative models of care and patient satisfaction, carer satisfaction and patients' quality of life, and the impact of alternative models on other services. We studied in more detail the care of patients dying in hospital and finally considered the differences between providing palliative care for patients with cancer or non-cancer diagnoses.

Method

A pre-defined protocol was followed in order to undertake a rigorous and comprehensive review of the literature from the UK, North America, Europe, and Australasia. Both comparative and descriptive studies were included. Searches were carried out in a range of electronic databases; five journals were hand-searched for relevant articles; and a number of individuals and organizations were consulted to ensure coverage of all important literature.

Over 2000 documents were identified, of which 673 were relevant and were reviewed. Essential data were extracted from each article in a common format, and then collated in a computer database. Checklists were used to assess the quality of each paper reviewed. The findings from research which addressed each of the 10 research questions were synthesized in sections of the report, supported where appropriate by tables of summary data from relevant papers.

Results

Most of the papers retrieved were small scale descriptions of local services, uncontrolled evaluations, or statements of opinion. There were few comparative trials of reasonable quality. The considerable difficulties of conducting research in the field of palliative care were evident. Much research came from the US, and may be of limited applicability to the UK.

Need for and provision of palliative care

There has been considerable expansion in provision of palliative care services in the UK in the last 30 years. The vast majority of patients receiving palliative care have cancer, and most evaluations have been in this group of patients. However, cancer deaths are exceeded by patients dying from stroke, neurological disease, heart failure, and AIDS. The process of dying for these patients is less predictable, but they may have unmet needs and poor symptom control and may benefit from palliative care. They may require a different emphasis in the provision of services. There is evidence that many patients' needs are not met in terms of place of death, with most patients wishing to die at home but less than one third doing so, mainly because of poor symptom control. Only half of the patients dying at home from cancer currently receive the support of a palliative care team or specialist nurse.

Models of care

The range of alternative models of palliative care is presented, with reference to descriptions and evaluations of each form of care. The importance of considering each model in the context of the different healthcare systems in different countries is highlighted. Although there are several descriptions and evaluations of hospital support teams and home care support teams, there are few evaluations of out-patient services, day care, hospice at home, or the potential effectiveness of non-specialist palliative care provided by the primary healthcare team. Evaluations of free-standing hospices are mainly dated and methodologically weak. The role of volunteers in palliative care has not been sufficiently evaluated.

Costs

The considerable investment in the expansion of palliative care services has not been accompanied by evidence of cost-effectiveness in the UK. In particular, the costs and benefits of home care supported by specialist palliative care teams versus in-patient hospice care have not been sufficiently addressed. Evidence from the US suggests that supported care at home provides a popular service, and is at least as effective as in-patient care at considerably lower cost. However, the relevance of these findings to the UK cannot be assumed.

Nursing skill-mix

A large number of surveys and descriptive studies were found. However, there was little useful evidence available to draw conclusions about different levels of nursing skill-mix, or the cost-effectiveness of clinical nurse specialists. Rigorous evaluation of this expanding workforce is clearly needed.

Patient and carer satisfaction

There is evidence from a number of studies that consumers are more satisfied with all types of palliative care, whether provided in in-patient units or in the community, than with care in general hospitals. The experiences and wishes of patients with cancer or non-cancer disease may differ, and more research is needed on consumer priorities for non-cancer diseases. Some studies highlighted difficulties with the care of dying patients in the community, although these findings were less clear than for hospitals.

Quality of life

There is some evidence that in-patient palliative care provides better pain control than home care or conventional hospital care. This is an important result, but is based on old research and needs confirmation. The research on palliative home care teams and co-ordinating nurses has demonstrated limited impact on quality of life over conventional care for patients dying at home. This negative finding may be due to the limitations of the assessment tools used. There is a need for a large and definitive study to provide clear evidence about whether further investment in these services can be justified in terms of impact on quality of life or symptom control.

Implications of alternative models of care for different sectors of the palliative care

The provision of specialist palliative care services appears to act as an additional service, rather than providing a substitute for existing services. As additional components of a complete specialist palliative care service are put in place, the total workload increases. Where in-patient palliative beds are provided the number of patients dying at home decreases, rather than fewer patients dying in hospital. Home care support services have not been shown to increase the proportion of patients dying at home.

Improving the care of patients dying in hospital

There is a paucity of evidence about the best forms of care for patients dying in hospital. Methodological difficulties are considerable. There is some evidence that hospice support teams may promote better symptom control, but research is needed on the efficacy of in-patient palliative care units, day hospitals, and the role of the clinical nurse specialist.

The relationship between models of care in cancer and other diseases

The similarities and differences in providing palliative care for patients with cancer and other diseases are discussed. Although the literature on care for AIDS patients is growing, there is little research about the needs of other groups, particularly those with renal failure, motor neurone disease, and dementia.

Conclusion

Despite the large quantity of literature examined there were few clear answers to any of the questions we addressed. There remains a need for both large scale research to provide clear answers about key questions, such as the value of home care support teams or the cost-effectiveness of in-patient hospice care, and also for small scale local research to assess new initiatives. Priority areas for research include:

- The palliative care needs of patients with non-cancer diagnoses.
- Whether or not home palliative care support teams and hospital support teams improve aspects of care other than patient satisfaction.
- The cost-effectiveness of in-patient palliative care in free-standing hospices in comparison with conventional hospital care and intensive home care support.
- The implications of the Calman–Hine report (Expert Advisory Group on Cancer 1995) for palliative care services for patients with cancer.
- The role of day hospitals.
- The costs and benefits arising from the clinical nurse specialist role in hospital.
- Options for improving palliative care in nursing homes and long-term care.
- Drug therapy and prescribing decisions in palliative care.
- Improving communication with carers.
- The development of psychosocial counselling and support as part of palliative care.
- The development of teams and shared process between primary and secondary care.
- The role of volunteers and self-help groups
- The role of family doctors in palliative care and ways of improving their ability to care.
- Evaluation of educational initiatives about palliative care for non-specialist staff.

2

Background

NICK BOSANQUET

Palliative care is as old as human compassion, but as an organized research-based field of care it dates back only 40 years. Beginning in the UK with the hospice movement and the inspiration of Cicely Saunders, palliative care now takes different forms and is based in different situations in home and in hospital. It is now a worldwide movement with great potential for improving care through initiatives which are relatively low in cost and feasible in terms of the human, therapeutic, and technical resources. Much of the treatment base in effective drugs is well established with morphine and its derivatives. In palliative care there is no need to yearn for breakthroughs round the corner: rather the problem is often one of frustration at goals which seem both tantalizingly close and frustratingly unattainable. Above all, the aim of a good death in which quality of life is maintained and if possible enhanced during the final phase of life still seems far off.

This critical literature review takes place at a time of change and challenge in palliative care. There is change in the funding outlook for health services among OECD members with a shift towards budgetary controls, slow growth in funding, and rationing of service all creating a difficult environment for any new area of care. There is the challenge of demographic change which will alter and increase the challenge to palliative care. The typical palliative care client of the future will no longer be the younger patient with cancer, let alone the consumptive heroine of *La Bohème*. The more typical patient will be elderly and have significant co-morbidity as well as possible cognitive problems. The diagnosis may often be one of cancer as well—but the challenge to care will be more long drawn out and may involve more kinds of support. The implications for healthcare costs will also be far greater: as any increase in institutional care at the end of life will add significantly to total cost through increased spending on nursing home or hospital admissions. At the same time expectations of better care will be improving and there will be more pressure to improve service to carers.

In this environment there will be greater impetus to seek new models of care. There is already some international divergence—perhaps more in this field than in almost any other of healthcare. The hospice building has become familiar in the UK but is much more rare in the US and virtually unknown in most of mainland Europe. There may well be pressures to improve palliative care much more within mainstream services rather than as a specialized additional service. Palliative care now faces a period of review and reassessment and there can be little complacency about access and quality as it is at present in most health systems.

Developments within the UK show how these new challenges have already begun to emerge in the 1990s. The first generation problem was about winning funding and support for specific projects where it was often simpler to raise capital spending for buildings. The next generation of problems will be about establishing a process so that all who need effective help across the whole range of conditions can get it—finding ways of enhancing and supporting quality of life in the last phase for many more people. Some of the new agendas in the UK may illustrate the challenges which palliative care is likely to face.

The range of services on offer is now far more varied and more complex than was the case even 5 years ago, covering hospice, hospice at home, home care teams, and hospital-based palliative care teams. Funders and managers are now faced with many more options for developing services. There is also more experience with defining contracts for access and quality in local services and a new level of concern about effectiveness and value for money.

There are new issues about how to develop partnership between specialist palliative care and care given by non-specialists, such as family doctors and community nurses. Specialist palliative care is now a national network available in most places, but many patients needing palliative care will still be receiving it from non-specialists. There is a new challenge in local development of the care process.

The role of carers is increasing with reduced length of hospital stay and more emphasis on care at home during terminal illness. At the same time, the role of nursing homes, especially in extreme old age, has increased, thus increasing the need for partnership between the private and public sectors.

The reorganization of acute services and concerns about quality are putting new pressures on terminal care in hospital. There are more demands for choice at the end of life.

The reorganization of cancer services is increasing the role of palliative care. In part this involves a movement towards a hub and spoke model of service: but it also involves a change in the process of care to increase the role of palliative care.

Our critical literature review aims to contribute to this process of reassessment and change—to a new phase of development. The last two decades were about projects with a focus on hospitals and teams of specialist nurses. The next phase is likely to be about networks and the use of IT and management focus to develop individual care programmes. Palliative care services for patients with AIDS-related disease have shown the creative potential for home based services and care programmes.

Our review aims to provide evidence on these development issues for the future and we have particularly tried to do this in an international context. This is perhaps the first attempt to document the development of palliative care as a worldwide movement. The programmes have developed so that there is now the potential for accelerated learning through international contact.

3

Aims and objectives

The overall aim for this book was to identify the most appropriate and cost-effective model of service delivery and level of provision of palliative care services. Within this general aim, 10 key questions were identified, which formed a framework for this review, and are referred to as Questions 1–10 throughout the review:

Question 1 What is the current *pattern of use* of services for palliative care, with particular respect to changing historical trends, geographical variation, and accessibility to patients?

Question 2 What is the current *level of need* for palliative care? What needs are there for different types of care, for different diseases and different patient groups, and at different stages of illness? This includes consideration of the different problems, both pain and non-pain, that require palliative care.

Question 3 What *models* for palliative care services have been proposed or developed in the UK, Europe, North America, and Australia?

Question 4 What evidence is available about the *costs and benefits* of various models of palliative care?

Question 5 What is the appropriate *skill-mix in palliative care nursing* in terms of specialist and general nursing skills? What are the costs and benefits associated with the clinical nurse specialist role in palliative care?

Question 6 What is known about *patient and carer preference* for, and satisfaction with, different types of palliative care?

Question 7 What is the impact of different models of care on *patients' quality of life*, psychological well-being, and motivation?

Question 8 What are the *implications* of alternative models of service delivery for different sectors of the palliative care network, (e.g. primary care, social services, Macmillan nurses) and for the wider use of resources (e.g. prescribing expenditure, social security, and the personal finances of patients and carers)?

Question 9 How can different models of organization or bed utilization improve the care of *patients dying in hospital*?

Question 10   What is the relationship between models of palliative care in cancer and palliative care in other diseases such as AIDS?

4

Conduct of the review

CHRIS SALISBURY

Systematic approach

The overall aim for this review was to identify and evaluate all published work which was relevant to the 10 previously listed questions in a rigorous and systematic manner. The questions were wide ranging, and not all of the issues were amenable to experimental trials. The review therefore included both qualitative and quantitative research with a wide variety of outcome measures.

A methodology of systematic reviews has been developed to compare similar trials addressing one specific research question. It usually involves synthezising the results of comparable experimental studies. This approach is not entirely applicable to the topics covered in this review. However, the principles of using explicit methods to identify and appraise the literature, exhaustive attempts to identify a comprehensive bibliography, structured extraction and analysis of data, and rigorous attempts to minimum bias all remain relevant, and are followed in this review.

Inclusion criteria

There was a two-stage process of inclusion. Firstly, there were several overall criteria:

- studies conducted in Europe, North America, Israel, and Australasia.
- studies involving palliative care for any disease
- both male and female patients of any age
- literature published in English, French, German, or Italian
- studies published since 1980 (It became apparent during the review that several important papers had been published in the

late 1970s. Such papers were included but comprehensive searches were not made of pre-1980 literature.)

Secondly, papers were included if they were relevant to one or more of the 10 research questions. For each question there were specific inclusion criteria determining the type of material to be reviewed:

Questions 1–3 Descriptive studies and analyses of available data.

Question 4 Primary studies which involved an assessment of costs and benefits from a particular model of palliative care. This included comparative and descriptive studies.

Question 5 Analyses of the relationship between alternative models of nursing in palliative care and workload, cost, nurse job satisfaction, reduced patient morbidity, increased patient functional ability, patient or carer satisfaction.

Question 6 Experimental or descriptive studies of models of palliative care which used measures of patient or carer satisfaction, preference or opinion as an end-point.

Question 7 Experimental and descriptive studies which considered the impact of models of palliative care on patients' quality of life.

Question 8 Any document which addressed the wider implications of alternative models of palliative care on other sectors of the health or social services. This included effects on charitable groups, social services provision, primary care, and acute hospitals of changes in the provision of care.

Question 9 Analyses of studies which considered the impact of different models of operation within hospitals on provision of palliative care.

Question 10 Documents describing the relationship between provision of, or need for, palliative care for patients with cancer, in relation to the need for care in other diseases such as AIDS and chronic neurological diseases.

The above criteria for the type of material to be included are quite general. It became clear during early examination of the literature that there were very few studies carried out using experimental methodologies and hardly any issues which had been addressed by more than one comparable experimental study. It was therefore necessary to include a wide range of types of research in the review.

Exclusion criteria

The general aim was to identify scientific research, both experimental and descriptive. Previous literature reviews were also valuable sources of information. It became apparent that the volume of literature was large, but that a large proportion of the available documents were of little value for this review. The following exclusion categories were developed:

- personal opinions and commentaries
- ethical, legal or religious issues in palliative care
- individual case histories
- education in palliative care
- history of palliative care provision
- development of research instruments (e.g. the development of quality of life measures)
- articles about cancer services generally, not primarily about palliative care.

In addition individual reviewers in some cases developed specific exclusion criteria within each of the 10 questions in order to focus the review and to eliminate material of limited relevance. Where such question-specific criteria occur they are described at the beginning of each chapter.

Definitions

The following definitions were used, based on those of the National Council for Hospice and Specialist Palliative Care Services (Wiles 1994). Similar definitions are to be found in the report from the Standing Medical and Nursing Advisory Committees (1992).

Palliative care is the active total care of patients and their families by a multiprofessional team when the patient's disease is no longer responsive to curative treatment.

Palliative care services is a broad term which covers provision in both community and inpatient settings. Services may be NHS or voluntary, multiprofessional or uniprofessional; and may be provided by individuals or teams. Some services will meet the definition of specialist palliative care services, others may not; they are all staffed by professionals who have extensive experience and/or additional training in aspects of palliative care, some up to specialist level.

Specialist palliative care services are those services with palliative care as their core speciality.

Terminal care is an important part of palliative care and usually refers to the management of patients during their last few days or weeks or even months of life from a point at which it becomes clear that the patient is in a progressive state of decline.

Hospice and **hospice care** refer to a philosophy of care rather than a specific building or service. The terms are generally avoided in the discussion in this report but are used in relation to buildings or organizations which refer to themselves in this way.

The above definitions are used in the UK. However, it is important to note that research from other countries may use these terms differently. This is particularly the case for North American research where the term 'hospice care' is used in relation to palliative care in whatever setting, and often refers to home-based care.

Sources of data

We identified documents to be reviewed in a number of ways. Sources of data included electronic and paper databases, registers of current research, reference lists and bibliographies, hand-searches of previous issues of medical journals, and a consultation process involving individuals and organizations.

Computer-based databases

The databases used were:

- Medline
- Embase
- Cochrane library
- Index of Scientific and Technical Proceedings
- SIGLE (Index of grey literature)

- NHS Project Research System
- Cancerlit
- Health Planning and Administration
- DHSS data.

Paper-based databases

- European Directory of Palliative Care Research
- Index of *Palliative Medicine* journal, provided by St Christopher's Hospice. This journal has only been referenced by Medline since 1993.

Hand searching

An initial search in Medline produced a draft bibliography. This was sorted by journal, to determine the five journals which had published most identified papers. These five journals were:

- *Hospice Journal*
- *Palliative Medicine*
- *Journal of Palliative Care*
- *Cancer Nursing*
- *Oncology Nursing Forum.*

The issues of the above journals for the previous five years (1992–96 inclusive) were hand-searched to identify any papers which had not already been found.

Current research

The following major funding organizations were asked to provide information about relevant projects which they were currently or had recently funded:

- NHS Project Register
- Cancer Research Council
- Medical Research Council
- Imperial Cancer Research Fund
- Wellcome Trust.

Reference lists

The reference lists of all articles that had been retrieved were scrutinised to identify further relevant studies.

Consultation

After the electronic literature searches had been conducted, several organizations were sent the preliminary bibliography. They were asked about:

- the comprehensiveness of the bibliography
- any missing studies they were aware of, particularly unpublished work or research in progress
- other sources of data, for example conferences which had not published proceedings, or journals or reports which were not indexed
- whether they held bibliographic or reference lists which might include studies of interest to this review.

The organizations which were contacted are listed in Appendix A.

In addition, several individual researchers were contacted. The *European Directory of Palliative Care Research* lists individuals and organizations who are active in palliative care research. Using this directory the individuals listed in Appendix B were asked to provide bibliographies of their research, and to inform us of any other material that may not be routinely available.

The advisory group

An expert advisory group was established to oversee the direction of the project and to take part in conducting the review. The group included representatives with expertise in palliative medicine, health economics, health policy, primary care, and nursing. Each member of this group took initial responsibility for one or more sections of the review.

Development of the search strategy

Initial literature searches were conducted in the electronic database

Medline using combinations of Mesh headings. These searches provided several thousand references, most of which were clearly irrelevant. Considerable difficulties were found in devising a search strategy which was sufficiently sensitive to identify all important material, yet specific enough to produce a manageable and relevant list. An examination of the indexing of the most important identified papers led us to the conclusion that a Mesh-based strategy would not be possible, and that it would be necessary to restrict the search using combinations of keywords. This did, however, lead to the risk of omitting important papers if they had imaginative titles and no recorded abstract in Medline. This risk was to some extent minimized by the wide range of free text words included, careful choice of words and use of 'wild-card' search strings, and the use of several search strategies. Eventually a main strategy was devised, as shown in Appendix C.

This strategy was devised for use with Silver Platter in Medline, and it identified 874 articles by the March 1997 update. As far as possible the same strategy was then replicated with all the other electronic databases, allowing for the fact that different databases used different indexing systems.

In addition, a series of searches were carried out in Medline, designed specifically to identify papers relevant to each research question, and a further search was carried out specifically to identify existing literature reviews.

Initial assessment of titles and abstracts

All references were examined from their titles and abstracts and allocated to one or more question numbers, or were coded as irrelevant or excluded (using the categories previously described). Those papers marked as irrelevant or excluded were double checked by another member of the review team.

Table 4.1 summarizes the papers which were identified and retrieved from all sources of data previously described

Data extraction

Data extraction forms were designed to allow the structured

Table 4.1   Numbers of papers identified and retrieved from all sources of data

Category	Number
Documents relevant, retrieved, and analysed	673
Documents relevant, but irretrievable	145
Documents initially thought relevant but when retrieved found to be irrelevant or excluded	129
Documents coded as irrelevant/excluded from their titles and abstracts and not retrieved	1282
Total number of documents identified	2229
Total number of documents reviewed	802

recording of important information about each document. This information included:

- research question number
- paper title and reference details
- country
- year in which data collected
- setting
- subjects
- disease type
- study design
- brief key points for general non-experimental/observational papers.

For experimental or observational studies, details were recorded of:

- the intervention or comparison
- the number of groups including controls
- the total number of subjects, and in each group
- the duration of the intervention
- the follow-up interval
- outcome measures

- details of randomization—unit of allocation/method of randomization
- measurement tools
- results
- cost of intervention and cost-effectiveness
- key conclusions
- comments about the strengths and weaknesses of the study.

Assessment of the quality of papers

All reviewers were provided with a series of checklists, to aid them in evaluating studies of different types (see Appendix D). These checklists were used by the reviewers to inform their comments about the strength and weaknesses of the studies, recorded in the final field of the data extraction form.

Data synthesis

Each reviewer produced a narrative report which synthesized the results of the papers they had evaluated, addressing one of the research questions. Where applicable they devised tables which compared and contrasted the results of similar studies, using the summary information collected in the extraction forms.

The variety of research methodologies and outcomes described in the identified papers was extremely wide. There were few instances where papers were directly comparable. It was therefore not appropriate to score papers formally according to their research quality or to carry out any statistical synthesis of research from a combination of primary studies. However, the concept of a hierarchy of evidence, whereby some research methodologies are accepted as more robust than others, was used in reaching conclusions in each section of the report, with more weight being given to well-conducted, controlled studies.

5

Problems of conducting research in palliative care

EMMA K. WILKINSON

Scope of research

The scope of research is bound by the definition of palliative care. Palliative care is the total active care of the patient when curative treatment is no longer responsive (Johnston and Abraham 1995). This care aims to address the 'whole patient', including his or her physical, mental, spiritual, and psychosocial needs (Wilkes *et al.* 1991). Care should extend beyond the patient to the families in providing care and bereavement support. The scope of research is therefore wide. As well as the need for research in the areas outlined, there is also a need for research into the management and organization of services (Twycross and Dunn 1994).

In practice, scientific evidence is hard to find in palliative care (Wilkes *et al.* 1991). The nature of dying is a complex, ever-changing process which makes the design and implementation of research particularly prone to certain problems and pitfalls. Palliative care for the dying is also a sensitive area to investigate and ethical considerations are paramount. All research should be based on the principles of respect for autonomy of participants, avoiding harm, justice, and benefit to participants (Crowther *et al.* 1995).

General research methods

Dying is a complex, dynamic process which changes with time. Given the complexities of dying, robust research methods are needed to permit meaningful collection and interpretation of data from research studies. As such, there is a need for studies of longitudinal design because these have a higher likelihood of monitoring such processes more effectively.

Qualitative research methods, such as ethnographic studies, non participant observation, case studies, interviewing (using open-ended questions), or diary studies are beneficial in obtaining data on subjective experience or observable data. However, careful attention needs to be given to issues of reliability and the potentially limited generalizability of results.

Quantitative research methods may provide greater assurance of reliability than qualitative methods. Examples of quantitative research methods include surveys or questionnaires involving closed responses. These methods may be employed in experimental or quasi-experimental intervention studies which utilize clearly defined outcome measures. The advantages of clearly defined outcome measures include the minimization of potential researcher bias in the interpretation of results and also in the testing of hypotheses.

Instrumentation

Instruments employed should be capable of valid and reliable measurement. The use of validated instruments is advocated wherever possible. Although many validated instruments are available for measuring symptoms, quality of life, and other outcomes, most have been designed for use in clinical settings other than palliative care. Such instruments may not be responsive enough to detect changes relevant in a palliative care setting. For example, measurements derived from the Karnosfsky Performance Status Scale for functional status have been criticised for providing crude measurements which do not reflect actual occurrences (Twycross and Dunn 1994). A low score on this scale may reflect the fact that a patient is bedridden, but may mask the fact that the patient is still socially and emotionally engaged.

Data collection

Data in a palliative care setting can be difficult to obtain. Indeed, patients requiring palliative care are likely to be physically weak and as they approach death, further physical deterioration and sometimes cognitive impairment occurs. Patients may lack the energy or concentration to complete surveys or questionnaires, and follow-up research is not guaranteed. Some may drop out due to death or severe illness (Moons *et al.* 1994). In general, as death approaches, fewer patients become available for participation in research. Not only has attrition proved a key problem in palliative care research, but recruitment of patients has also proved problematic. For example, McWhinney *et al.* (1994) experienced difficulty in recruiting patients for participation in a randomized controlled trial, as some health professionals perceived it unethical to deny some patients the right to treatment or 'special conditions' The fact that not all patients with terminal disease need palliative care should be considered in the design of randomized controlled trials for the results to be meaningful.

An alternative to relying on patients to give information is to use proxies to provide assessments. Proxies may include friends, relatives, or health professionals. Although proxies may be more willing participants and easier to interview, the validity of their views in terms of representing the experiences of the patients is questionable. The extent to which the views of 'proxies' diverge from those of patients is still not fully understood (Fakhoury *et al.* 1997). Retrospective assessments made by relatives or friends may be affected by the process of grief. Higginson *et al.* (1994a) found that in comparison with prospective assessments, bereaved family members' memories of symptoms and pain were polarized after death of patients. Although prospective or retrospective information provided by other proxies such as health professionals or independent assessors may be less biased, it may also be limited in content and more costly to obtain (Twycross and Dunn 1994).

A further alternative to relying on information from a small number of patients is to collect data from patients across multiple sites or from single-case experiments which measure specific changes in patients over time (Twycross and Dunn 1994). This, however, raises the problem of ensuring reliable data collection from multiple sites.

Assessment of outcome measures

Outcome measures aim to measure the effects of palliative care services or certain intervention(s) on certain aspects of care. As the objectives of such interventions are likely to be unique to palliative care, so the outcome measures should reflect the special concerns within palliative care. Examples of general areas used as outcome measures include quality of life, quality of death, psychological status, personal finances, and symptom and pain control. It is notable that the aspects of care relevant to some outcome measures have not been supported by a clear consensus either within or beyond palliative care, for example, quality of life measures (Higginson 1995a).

For research in any healthcare field, there are potential difficulties in the assessment outcome measures as the relationship between the intervention and health status is an imperfect one. This is due to the presence of psychological, social and environmental factors which may influence the outcome. Research in the field of palliative care is of no exception. Outcome measures may be subject to threats to internal and external validity. For example, even randomized controlled trials which provide baseline measures and a control group against which to measure the effects of experimental treatment, and which eliminate bias through randomization, have failed to provide firm, scientific evidence, owing to threats to internal validity (e.g. McWhinney *et al.* 1994, Rinck *et al.* 1995). Various threats to the internal validity of research designs are outlined below.

Attrition

The problem of attrition is one of the biggest problems faced by researchers as it results in difficulties in achieving an adequate sample size to make it possible to assess the effectiveness of the intervention with any certainty. Attrition may change the composition of groups, making comparisons between groups and generalizations more difficult.

Heterogeneity of participants

In any group of patients, total homogeneity is unattainable. This problem is more marked in groups of dying patients, when there is a scarcity of patients available for inclusion in research. As such, the resulting heterogeneity of case-mix in terms of variation in aetiologies, prognoses, and symptoms will serve to diminish the statistical certainty of outcome measures.

Unreliable, inaccurate or crude instrumentation

Outcome measures developed in other clinical settings may not be sensitive to the changes which occur within a palliative care environment and may lack appropriateness, for example they may be too long for participants to complete. Such instruments are likely to be poor indicators of effect (Wilkes *et al.* 1991).

Attribution of change

Owing to the natural deterioration of patients, the certainty of attributing change to the research intervention or specific type of care is particularly difficult to determine. Since there is often more than one professional group or set of individuals providing care, attributing changes to the specific intervention is also difficult. For example, dilution of effect occurred when a group of hospice patients in a randomized controlled trial were exposed to the conditions of the other 'hospital group' as they were cared for in general wards when hospice beds were full (Kane *et al.* 1984).

Timing

Patients may experience significant fluctuations in pain, mood, and psychological state on approaching death, which can make it difficult to collect valid data reliably reflecting the experiences of patients (Wales *et al.* 1983). The timing of the data collected is crucial in detecting these changes and when they occur in relation to any intervention (Wilkes *et al.* 1991).

Variation in assessments made by assessors

The impact of the assessors, such as patients, relatives, or health professionals should also be considered in the assessment of outcome measures wherever appropriate.

Generalization of results

Caution in generalizing the findings to other settings or groups is necessary for several reasons. The following are examples of potential threats to external validity if not adequately controlled.

Self-selection bias

If no measures are taken to control for the potential self-selection of patients, the results may be based on subjects who are not representative (Dush and Cassileth 1985).

Responses not reflecting participants' real opinions

Respondents may feel under greater pressure to provide socially desirable answers to sensitive questions (Fakhoury *et al.* 1997) and the reluctance of recipients of care to criticize providers of care is well documented (Kelson 1995). Pressure to provide socially desirable answers may be heightened in face-to-face interviews, compared to self-administered questionnaires. Also, participants' responses may be altered as a function of being observed and may not reflect the respondents' real opinions (Hawthorne effect). Alternatively, strong positive, first impressions of one aspect of care may distort consumers' views of other aspects of care, which can lead to positive over-generalizations (halo effect).

Differences between sites

Making meaningful comparisons between the quality of care provided in different sites may also prove problematic. This is partially due to the fact that differences between institutions are not clear (Seale 1989). For example, some institutions providing palliative care services may be considered 'pioneering centres' and may have been the focus of many studies, such as St Christopher's Hospice. The extent to which findings derived from 'pioneering centres' can be meaningfully compared to other institutions whose standards are less well known is questionable.

Differences between countries

Direct comparisons between research findings derived from palliative care settings in different countries may prove complicated because of cultural differences, and differences in the provision of palliative care services. Differences in the financial arrangements in funding palliative care services have led to the development of unique systems of care in the UK and North America. The structure of these services differs in fundamental ways; for example, primary care services in the UK are more developed, therefore the role of home care teams in Britain is to 'support' primary healthcare teams, rather than to 'provide' care independently. Finding evidence that a system of care works well in one country may not indicate in itself that it will work well in another.

Utility

The utility of merely considering the 'effect' achieved by intervention studies has been questioned (Higginson and McCarthy 1989). To ensure greater utility of results, it is important to consider and describe the full context in which the results were obtained (Higginson and McCarthy 1989). Consideration of the 'full context' means examining what kinds of interventions took place, their possible combinations, and also the circumstances in which they took place. Further consideration should also be paid to the types of participants and their characteristics, as well as the researchers' aims and concerns.

Relevance of methodological issues to this systematic literature review

The fact that firm scientific evidence is difficult to find in palliative care has meant that a large proportion of the studies we reviewed were non-experimental, descriptive papers or those based mainly on expert opinion (as opposed to experimental studies with findings supported by firm evidence). The methodological issues raised in this section, including difficulties regarding data collection, assessment of outcome measures, instrumentation, generalization, and utility of results, were common limitations of the literature we reviewed.

To address concerns regarding the potential limitations of some studies, we have presented the details of the most reliable, informative studies in the context in which the research took place. These details are given in a tabular format within the relevant chapters. We have also discussed the shortcomings as well the reliability of evidence derived from the research studies. In this way, we aimed to maximize the utility of our results as well as to present an accurate, balanced view of the main research findings on cost-effective models of palliative care.

II

The 10 questions

Question 1 ....

Patterns of use of service

NICK BOSANQUET

What is the current pattern of use of services for palliative care with particular reference to changing historical trends, geographical variation and accessibility to patients?

UK

The development of palliative care started in the late 1960s from a position where palliative care was provided by non-specialists in hospitals, general practice, and community nursing. In the 1970s and 1980s the main emphasis was on the development of specialist services, first in hospices and then in home care teams and hospitals.

Addington-Hall and McCarthy (1995a) provide good evidence on the pattern of service in the early 1990s based on a sample of 20 health districts in the UK. Of the achieved sample of 2074 cancer deaths, 14% took place in hospices, 50% in hospitals, 29% in own homes and 7.3% in nursing homes: 60% had care from a district nurse and 29% from a hospice home care or specialist nurse. The level of specialist service to non-cancer patients was low.

Reasons for seeking palliative care

There is little direct evidence on what motivates patients who seek different levels of palliative care, but some indirect evidence on why home-based palliative care breaks down.

Thorpe (1993) provides a review of the reasons for use of hospital admission in the last stage. They include failure to control symptoms, excessive nursing and—most commonly—stress on relatives or carers. Most of the focus has been, however, on symptom control rather than on these social and holistic elements. Addington-Hall and McCarthy (1995a) use symptom control as one of their main indicators, and a local study by Hinton (1994b) suggests that the more social areas have received less attention. According to Hinton 'the awareness of dying and coping attitudes of patients at first interview were better indicators of which patients were likely to die at home than the symptoms which they volunteered at that point'.

Service patterns

Detailed information is available on service patterns by hospices and associated home care teams. By 1997 there were 223 in-patient hospice units (Hospice Information Service 1997b). Average length of stay in hospices was falling with a median length of stay of 14 days. There were 234 units providing day care at the beginning of 1997. The most common number of places was 10 and the average attendance was 1½ days per week. There were 7500 places a week.

Less information was available on hospital support services. There were 176 services providing a hospital support nurse. The hospital-based services had higher caseloads, with many nurses seeing 250 or more new patients per year. In 1993 hospices had 56 000 admissions (Eve and Smith 1996). Specialist home care services seemed to follow two different models. In one, direct involvement with patients and families to provide support monitoring and occasionally practical nursing care formed a major part of the work. In the other a more distinctive specialist role was developed where advising and training other professionals in the community and in hospital took precedence over direct patient contact although this was maintained (Boyd 1994).

The original impetus to the growth of the hospice movement came in the late 1960s with the foundation of St Christopher's Hospice. The first period of growth concentrated on in-patient services in the 1970s. The growth was mainly driven by local enthusiasm and local fund-raising and the pattern of development did not lead to an even pattern of access. A survey by Lunt and Hillier in 1980 showed that there were 58 in-patient units, 32 home care teams, and 8 hospital support teams. Of the 58 units, 37 were outside the

information services
gwasanaethau gwybodaeth

Cancer Research Wales Library
Llyfrgell Ymchwil Cancr Cymru

With compliments
Gyda chyfarchion

Velindre Hospital, Whitchurch Cardiff, CF14 2TL Tel/Ffon: 029 20 316291
Ysbyty Felindre, Yr Eglwys Newydd, Caerdydd, CF14 2TL Fax/Ffacs: 029 20 316927
library@velindre-tr.wales.nhs.uk

31.07.09.

Rehoused with

Thanks.

CARDIFF
UNIVERSITY

PRIFYSGOL
CAERDYͰ

NHS and there were considerable differences in numbers of places between regions.

Lunt showed in a later survey that the regional differences had begun to narrow, mainly as a result of a determined effort by one charity, the National Society for Cancer Relief (NSCR), to even up provision (Lunt 1985).

Wilkes (1984) provided some of the impetus for a further period of growth. His survey showed great difficulties for relatives, poor symptom control, and uncaring attitudes from some hospitals.

This survey confirms the inevitable tendency in any big service for a minority to deliver exceptionally good and another minority exceptionally bad care. We have for the first time attempted to quantify these proportions. Furthermore, although terminal care in the UK is several years ahead of the standards attained in some other western countries, there is still clearly room for improvement. It is only realistic to accept that most dying patients will feel weak, immobile, depressed, or anorexic to some degree: but that a high proportion of patients have ineffectively controlled pain, cough, dyspnoea, or insomnia is unsatisfactory, especially when only a third of them are routinely receiving opioids, and high doses are only rarely used (Wilkes 1984).

A good review by Taylor (1983) also defined some of the key issues for service development, including those of continuing independence or more integration with the NHS. Growth accelerated in the early 1990s as a result of greater availability of funding from NHS sources for capital development and more revenue support from local health authorities.

Access to care

There were concerns about access of patients from ethnic minorities to hospice care and that minority groups from different cultures might not find the hospice environment very welcoming (Hill and Penso 1995). There were also concerns about access to palliative care for patients with dementia. Few of these patients seemed to be getting palliative care at the moment, even though their symptoms made it likely that palliative care could have been highly relevant and appropriate. A retrospective study of patients with dementia showed that they experienced symptoms with a similar frequency to cancer patients but they experienced them for longer

(McCarthy *et al.* 1997a). A local survey of 10 hospices in the London area also showed low demand from patients with cardiac failure (Jones 1995).

In terms of immediate service use, most attention was on the issue of hospital admission in terminal care. One study showed a strong relationship between proportions dying at home and level of social deprivation with $r = -0.65$ for 44 wards in the London area from 1988–92. The range was from 5% who died at home in Kelfield ward (UPA Score 24) to 46% in Knightsbridge ward (UPA score 3) (Higginson *et al.* 1994b). By the 1990s one local survey showed there were differences of view between general practitioners and hospital doctors: general practitioners were much more likely to see terminal admissions to specialist units as having been inappropriate (Seamark *et al.* 1995). Concern was also being expressed about relative quality: 'At what point does increasing availability of specialist care start to de-skill other professionals?' (Regnard and Parker 1994).

Future challenges

Palliative care faced new challenges to improve services in the home and to provide a wider range of services including physio-therapy (Clark 1994). There were problems of pressure on unpaid carers and the fragmentation of paid care so that 'up to 25 different paid carers may visit a person's home during the course of the terminal illness' (Field and James 1993). There were criticisms of the variability and the lack of systematic relationship to local needs of the expanding services in day care. A survey of 12 units carried out by Higginson and Wilkes for Help the Hospices concluded that more evaluation was urgently required (Faulkner *et al.* 1993). The NHS reforms put pressure on many hospices to define their services (Malson *et al.* 1996). Thus by the 1990s there were new and growing concerns about access, quality and the organization of services.

The position of the hospices in relation to the NHS had changed: the service had become much more national, with a more even access, but many of the old problems still seemed to be causing concern even in the 1990s. The development of palliative care showed a cycle of concern leading to growth in services, but then renewed concern as the old problems seemed to recur.

USA

Patterns of service

The timing and development of the programme has been very different from that in the UK although the work of Dame Cicely Saunders has been a powerful inspiration in both countries.

The origins of palliative care in the USA date back to the early 1970s, when Dame Cicely Saunders came to Yale University in Connecticut to give a lecture to an audience composed of physicians, nurses, and community representatives on the care of patients for whom cure is no longer possible.

Cicely Saunders's message stimulated the imagination of the Yale community on the possibility of starting a hospice programme in Connecticut to demonstrate that, as Cicely Saunders had so eloquently described, people can die 'painlessly, peacefully and with dignity' (Magno 1992).

Funding issues around Medicare have been the major force in US development. The first US hospice was started in Connecticut in 1974 (Lukashok 1990). The American development has been mainly of three types:

- in-hospice care with an increasing emphasis on 'hospice at home' programmes
- palliative care units based in hospitals
- home care covering chronic as well as terminal illness.

In effect 'hospice' means a type of care in the US, whereas in the UK it usually refers to a building. A review carried out for the National Cancer Institute in 1990 showed that there were some 1700 hospices providing palliative care for over 200 000 patients of whom 85% died of cancer. A typical hospice is a small community-based or hospital-based programme that has a daily census of 22 patients and an average length of stay of 6 days and serves 124 patients a year. Thus the US programme reaches about 1 in 5 of the deaths from cancer in the US.

The development of hospice care up to 1990 is well charted by Magno (1992). The first hospice and five other demonstration projects were funded by the National Cancer Institute. In 1978 the Healthcare Financial Administration (HCFA) funded 23 selected hospice programmes and these were evaluated in the national

Hospice Study. In 1983 hospice care was made available to Medicare patients but under restrictive conditions which led to slower than expected growth in numbers covered. Continuing funding problems led hospices to shift towards home-based care and to reduce the number of in-patient beds. By the late 1980s hospice growth seemed to have reached a plateau. Physician attitudes were seen as a continuing problem, with slow development of a specialty in palliative medicine and lack of awareness or outright opposition by other physicians. Roussea (1994) and McCue (1995) discuss these barriers to communication:

Many physicians fail to understand the tenet of hospice care and erroneously presume hospice programmes help patients die (Rousseau 1994).

The medicalization of dying is a pernicious trend that runs counter to several powerful societal changes and results in wasteful and bad medical care (Sun 1993).

Home care was much more available across the US in paediatric oncology: 85.9% of oncology centres were offering home care in 1984 (Lauer *et al.* 1986).

American perceptions and ideals after the first 15 years are well surveyed by Stoddard (1989) and by Lukashok (1990).

The work of Kubler Ross on death and dying has clearly been a more major influence than in the UK (Kubler Ross 1989). The American hospice movement has tended to stress holistic care, with a substantial use of volunteers and separation from mainline hospital programmes. Pre-Medicare developments of the programme are covered in numerous publications from the National Hospice Study by a team led by Mor at Brown University. Detailed studies showed that the availability of beds seemed to encourage admissions (Mor and Hiris 1983) and that home-based hospice patients had shorter periods of care than hospice-based ones (Mor *et al.* 1985).

The impact of Medicare

Bonham *et al.* (1987) report the impact of Medicare reimbursement on hospices in Kentucky in 1982–85. There was a substantial increase in admissions and by 1985 hospice care was covering 40% of cancer deaths. The percentage of hospice patients dying at home rose from 53% to 63% even though use increased among the elderly. Among all cancer patients only 23% died at home. On the other hand, a study of hospices in Pennsylvania in 1985–87 by Kriebel (1989) showed a reduced number of admissions and more emphasis on in-patient care. Magno (1992) stresses the major adjustment problems for hospices as a result of Medicare and shows how the hospice in south-eastern Michigan faced severe financial crisis and had to switch from in-patient to home care. Lukashok stresses how reimbursement through Medicare changes the identity and service provided by hospices:

By providing a hospice benefit under Medicare, the government has, in effect, defined what a hospice is. This legislation has succeeded in objectifying the hospice as a service, thereby specifying and credentialing the people who provide the service. It is particularly striking that a re-imbursement program that was intended to enhance the capacity of the terminally ill elderly to obtain a specific modality of care has fundamentally altered that modality of care. ... Cost savings will be marginal in the context of overall Medicare expenditures and are peripheral to the central programmatic concern which, from the broadest policy perspective, is not the future of hospice care in the United States, but rather the way in which the health system and its professionals provide care for terminally ill patients. The hospice is making its most lasting contribution in fostering and serving as a model for the incorporation into the system of a whole range of attitudes, techniques, and perspectives on the palliative care of the dying patient. And this process of influence has undoubtedly been stimulated and accelerated by the recognition of hospice care through the Medicare reimbursement benefit. (Lukashok 1990)

Carney *et al.* (1989) give a useful case study on the effect of Medicare. Patients in need of longer term care were switched to home healthcare and hospices were looking after sicker patients for shorter periods of time. In this case, in an urban area in the South West, the quantity of service measured in minutes per day increased by 40% and more of the service was given by registered nurses. Some hospitals were also inspired by the hospice movement to develop palliative care teams. Erle (1982) gives a case study for such a team at the New York Cornell Medical Center. Moinpour and Polissar (1989) show in Washington state that hospice availability was effective in 1980–85 in increasing numbers dying at home.

Developments for the future

Levy (1993) for the National Cancer Institute stresses the inadequate coverage of hospice programmes and the need to develop palliative care as a medical speciality. The American Geriatrics Society put forward principles for improving the care of dying patients and stressed that

'patients and families are presently faced with major financial obstacles in choosing palliative care while payment for continued highly technological care is readily available' (Sachs 1995)

There was also concern about the needs of patients with end-stage dementia. A national survey showed that fewer than 1% of hospice patients had a primary diagnosis of end-stage dementia and only 21% of hospices served such patients (Hanrahan and Luchins 1995a). There was concern about the lack of palliative care in nursing homes following earlier research by Wershow (1976) showing the important role of nursing homes in terminal care. Sager *et al.* (1988) also showed increased mortality in nursing homes in Wisconsin in the 1980s.

Parallel to the development of the hospices, there were controversies on the high costs of dying following the finding in 1984 that the 5.9% of Medicare enrolees who died in the year accounted for 27.9% of Medicare spending. These studies encouraged the development of home care services as a lower cost alternative to hospital treatment and also encouraged movement towards signing of living wills. Thus the focus for debate was on over use of high-tech care in the last stage of life rather than on lack of access to palliative care.

Europe

Apart from the UK, there was little interest either in hospice or in palliative care in most of mainland Europe. Albrecht (1990) reviews negative attitudes to hospices and financial barriers to home-based care in West Germany. There were also restrictions on the prescribing of opioids. In Italy there were some successful developments of local programmes for home-based care in Palermo (Mercadante and Mangione 1990) and Genoa (Costantini *et al.* 1993). In Sweden there was little interest in hospices but attempts to improve care for dying patients within the ordinary health system (Hjelmerus 1987). Surveys showed inadequate pain control in the Netherlands with development of palliative care programmes only in the 1990s (Zylicz

1996). The most active development was to be found in Catalonia (Gomez-Baptiste 1992). In response to the Who Global Project on palliative care, 30 home care teams were set up and there were training courses for family physicians. There was also special attention to the problems of AIDS patients in prisons.

Australia, Canada, and New Zealand

The hospice movement has developed strongly in South Australia. By 1990 South Australia had the highest coverage of any population in the world, with 56% of patients who died in 1990 having care from a hospice service. As in the UK, place of death was influenced by social factors. There were low proportions of deaths at home in country areas and within the city of Adelaide the proportions of deaths at home were 63.7% in the 'relatively more affluent Adelaide Southern urban and Tea Tree Gully sub-regions' (Roder *et al.* 1987). In other states in Australia, the emphasis was much more on improving services within the general hospitals. Malden *et al.* (1984) studied terminal care in Sydney in the early 1980s and stressed the need for improved palliative care in major hospitals. By the early 1990s Lefroy (1992) could comment that the separate development of these services was no longer desirable or necessary. Bradshaw (1993) reviews the wide range of services available in Western Australia.

Canada saw active development of palliative care within hospitals, as well as development of hospices following early inspiration by Dr Balfour Mount in Montreal. The growth up to the late 1980s is well surveyed by Hudson (1990). Most programmes were funded out of hospital global budgets. Muzzin *et al.* (1994) provide insight into the patient experience of cancer. New Zealand has also shown very substantial development with some hospices, but also more stress on hospital-based units. The New Zealand situation is well reviewed by Lichter (1990).

Developing countries

Without being able to carry out a comprehensive review, we report some interesting findings.

The WHO launched its global programme on palliative care against a background of evidence that 75% of cancer patients world-wide had untreated pain (Stjernsward 1988). Laudico (1993) records the first efforts to improve the situation in the Philippines. Yan Sun (1993) has carried out a trial of improved pain control in three cities of China against a background of late detection and poor palliation. Across the world there is a long way to go—even in countries with a history of development in palliative care—before the problems defined by the WHO are addressed.

Question 2

Need for palliative care

PETER J. FRANKS

What is the current level of need for palliative care?

When considering the current level of need one must define the patient groups in whom palliative care may be appropriate. In the past palliative care has often been restricted to patients suffering from terminal cancer, with hospice services dealing almost exclusively with these patients. However, there is a growing recognition that other diseases require periods of palliation. Higginson (1995b) recognizes three main disease categories which may require palliative care. These are broadly, cancer, non-malignant progressive diseases, and children's terminal illnesses (see Table 2.1).

Palliative care cannot be measured with commonly used outcome measures such as mortality or disability, but requires measurement of aspects which are important to patients with progressive disease and their families. It therefore deals with the quality of life, quality of death and dying, and the bereavement outcome. ... Clearly, outcomes may reflect positive or adverse events within the area of care; although most of the available outcome measures tend to measure the presence, absence or degree of problems, such as pain, anxiety, symptoms, rather than positive events such as fulfilment in life. (Higginson 1995b)

To estimate the need for palliative care two strategies may be adopted: epidemiological methods or the evaluation of health service use. The epidemiological approach uses the cause-specific mortality in diseases which are likely to benefit from palliative care services, and then relates this to the type and frequency of symptoms experienced by patients suffering from these terminal diseases. Health service use is an important means of evaluating need, in that it identifies patients who are within the services. It has the limitation that it does not assess unmet need which must then be evaluated

Table 2.1   Types of illness which may require palliative care (Higginson 1995b)

Types of illness	Main categories	
Cancer	Lung, trachea, bronchus Ear, nose, and throat Female breast Lymphatic Digestive tract Genitourinary Leukaemia haemopoetic	
Progressive non-malignant disease	Circulatory diseases:	– cardiovascular – cerebrovascular
	Respiratory diseases	
	Nervous system	– motor neurone disease – multiple sclerosis – dementia
	AIDS/HIV	
Children's terminal illnesses	Hereditary degenerative disorders Muscular dystrophy Cystic fibrosis	

by alternative means. We have examined both methods of need assessment, and report the results of both.

Epidemiological approach to needs assessment

Higginson (1995b) classifies patients into three categories:

- those who have a palliative care period prior to death
- those who had stable disease, with few symptoms followed by sudden death
- those who suffer from stable disease, but who might have periods of progression and symptoms, who would benefit from periods of palliative care followed by remission.

For patients suffering from cancer, the predicted progression most often falls into the first category. However, non-malignant disease quite often falls into the latter two categories, particularly circulatory diseases where death may follow a short symptomatic period.

Mortality statistics in England and Wales

Disease-specific mortality can be estimated from information supplied through death certificates, tabulated by the Office for National Statistics (formerly Office of Populations, Censuses and Surveys). The most recent figures available are for 1995 (Anonymous 1997). Although it is acknowledged that death certification includes many inherent inaccuracies in the causes of death (Gau and Diehl 1982), there is some evidence that the errors in certification are randomly distributed. Thus, although the individual certificate may not be a true reflection of the individuals cause of death, the overall disease specific mortality rates are accurate. Table 2.2 gives the death rates for causes which may require a period of palliation. Although cancer deaths are considered most often in palliative care services, it is clear that these make up only a proportion of all deaths which may have required palliative care. Deaths due to circulatory diseases are far more common than cancer deaths, though relatively few of these may include prolonged symptomatic periods requiring palliative care. To establish the importance of palliative care one must examine the frequency, duration, and intensity of symptoms in these diseases.

Assessing the symptoms of patients who have died

Two methods have been proposed to assess the prevalence of symptoms in patients in the terminal stages of a disease. Patients may be examined during their stay in specialist healthcare facilities, or relatives or healthcare professionals may be contacted following the patients' death to ascertain symptoms suffered prior to death. Both methods are problematic in providing accurate assessments for patient populations. In the former method, only patients attending a particular health facility are interviewed. It is generally acknowledged that patients who attend such units are atypical of the patient populations as a whole. To overcome this, random samples of

Table 2.2 Mortality statistics in England and Wales (Anonymous 1997). Values are deaths per million population

Age	Sex	Neoplasms	Circulatory diseases	Respiratory diseases	Nervous diseases	Congenital abnormalities
All	M	2831	4432	1549	174	26
	F	2543	4630	1782	191	25
<1	M	24	96	223	184	394
	F	28	76	165	127	351
1–4	M	34	12	20	32	47
	F	29	13	22	34	37
5–14	M	40	11	9	18	13
	F	31	8	11	12	16
15–24	M	59	37	22	45	14
	F	46	21	12	25	12
25–34	M	109	91	48	38	15
	F	141	59	26	28	11
35–44	M	334	401	98	54	15
	F	489	162	46	44	14
45–54	M	1338	1557	238	92	15
	F	1539	511	152	76	16
55–64	M	4503	5330	929	171	20
	F	3627	2041	630	140	22
65–74	M	12 073	16 345	4343	447	28
	F	7602	8454	2732	366	30
75–84	M	22 540	41 150	16 099	1443	64
	F	12 029	27 804	9130	975	46
85+	M	31 605	82 490	51 335	3103	79
	F	15 918	71 122	34 723	2126	54

patients who died from a particular cause may be identified through death certification. This method may produce a representative sample, but introduces errors due to proxy reporting of symptoms by a patient's relative or healthcare provider. There is evidence that carers overestimate the severity of symptoms compared with patients, and that general practitioners generally record fewer symptoms than hospital nurses, whereas relatives frequently record higher frequency of symptoms than the health professionals (Wilkes 1984). There is a clear need for prospective studies to accurately record symptoms in random samples of the patient populations.

Without such studies the assessment of need will be open to in-accuracies.

Prevalence of symptoms in patients suffering from terminal cancer

The prevalence of symptoms in patients with terminal cancer is given in Table 2.3. Clearly there is little consistency between different studies, probably reflecting differences in patient populations and the tools used to assess symptom frequency. In addition, different symptoms have been selected in different studies, as indicated by the number of cells with missing data. In some studies prevalence of vomiting and/or nausea have been combined (Cartwright 1991a, Boyd 1993, Hardy *et al.* 1994, Myers and Trotman 1995), and others have described other symptoms, which for the sake of clarity have been excluded here.

Pain is the most frequently investigated symptom in patients suffering from terminal illness. However, there is considerable vari-ation in its reported frequency, varying from 11% to 84% in differ-ent patient groups (Reuben *et al.* 1988, Coyle *et al.* 1990, Addington Hall *et al.* 1991, Cartwright 1991a, Boyd 1993, Hardy *et al.* 1994, Dudgeon *et al.* 1995, Hopwood and Stephens 1995, Myers and Trotman 1995, Zylicz 1996). This variation may be caused by meth-odological differences, not least the method of symptom ascertain-ment, selection of patients, and the use of proxy reporting. It is surprising that reported pain was highest in the random sample of patients. One would expect pain to be most severe in the most severe cases being treated by specialist units. However, similar levels have been reported in a random sample of 45 hospice service and 126 other cancer patients (Seale 1991b). In all, 93% hospice patients experienced pain compared with 80% of other cancer patients. In a review of the literature (Stjernsward 1988) it was estimated that moderate to severe pain occurs in 45–100% of patients with ad-vanced cancer, in whom it is inadequately managed in 20–40%.

Cancer pain relief is a ubiquitous but neglected public health problem. Every day more than three and a half million people suffer from cancer pain, but only a fraction receive treatment for it. Relatively simple and inexpensive methods of pain relief are available. Adequate pain relief is not reaching a great number of cancer patients in developed countries. In the developing countries, where more than half the world's cancer patients are

Table 2.3   Prevalence of symptoms in patients with terminal cancer

Study	Patients	Pain	Dyspnoea	Fatigue	Vomit	Nausea
Reuben *et al.* (1988)	mixed (*n* = 1592)	11	53	–	–	44
Cartwright (1991a)	random (*n* = 168)	84	47	–	–	–
Hardy *et al.* (1994)	mixed (*n* = 107)	67	28	–	–	–
Coyle *et al.* (1990)	mixed (*n* = 90)	34	28	52	–	13
Addington-Hall *et al.* (1991)	mixed (*n* = 80)	57	64	–	27	30
Dudgeon *et al.* (1995)	mixed (*n* = 75)	71	51	–	–	–
Boyd (1993)	mixed (*n* = 47)	36	38	–	–	–
Myers and Trotman (1995)	mixed (*n* = 32)	52	21	–	–	–
Site-specific studies						
Hopwood and Stephens (1995)	small cell lung cancer (*n* = 232)	45	87	88	20	38
Hopwood *et al.* (1991)	breast (*n* = 211)	–	–	–	–	–

and where most are incurable at the time of diagnosis, pain relief (often the only relevant humane alternative) by and large is not offered. (Stjernsward 1988)

Respiratory problems are also frequently cited in studies of terminal cancer patients, with prevalence varying from 21% to 64% with mixed cancer sites (Reuben *et al.* 1988, Coyle *et al.* 1990, Addington Hall *et al.* 1991, Cartwright 1991a, Boyd 1993, Hardy *et al.* 1994, Dudgeon *et al.* 1995, Myers and Trotman 1995). As expected, this is substantially higher (87%) in the patients suffering from lung cancer (Hopwood and Stephens 1995). Frequency of nausea varies in different studies from 13% to 44% (Reuben *et al.* 1988, Coyle *et al.* 1990, Addington Hall *et al.* 1991, Hopwood and Stephens 1995), and vomiting from 10% to 27% (Addington Hall *et al.* 1991, Hopwood and Stephens 1995). In studies where vomiting

(as percentages)

Sleep	Weak	Confused	Loss of appetite	Constipation	Incontinence	Anxiety	Depression
–	–	12	79	54	–	–	–
51	–	33	71	47	37	–	38
–	35	–	–	38	–	–	12
57	49	28	6	7	6	18	4
57	–	47	87	64	40	29	54
69	81	–	55	–	–	–	–
–	25	–	–	9	–	–	–
–	12	3	–	19	6	–	–
75	88	–	75	55	–	65	60
–	–	–	–	–	–	18	18

and nausea have been combined frequency ranges from 9% to 51% (Cartwright 1991a, Boyd 1993, Hardy *et al.* 1994, Myers and Trotman 1995).

Using the figures derived from the random sample (Cartwright 1991a) Higginson (1995) estimated that 2400 patients of the 2800 cancer deaths per million population would have experienced pain prior to their death, with 1300 patients would suffer breathing difficulties and 1400 would suffer from symptoms of vomiting or nausea.

Prevalence of symptoms in patients suffering from non-malignant terminal disease

A number of studies have investigated the prevalence of symptoms in cancer and non-cancer deaths combined (Wilkes 1984, Hockley *et al.*

1988, Cowley 1993, Lickiss *et al.* 1994), but only one random sample has examined symptoms in patients dying from non-cancer causes (Cartwright 1991a) (Table 2.4). Using these data on 471 non-cancer deaths it is clear that a lower proportion of these patients experienced pain (67%) than the cancer patients (87%), though there were still high proportions of patients who experienced respiratory problems (49%) and nausea/vomiting (27%). Using these data Higginson (1995) estimated that of 6900 patients with progressing non-malignant deaths per million population, 3400 would experience pain, 3400 would suffer from respiratory problems, and 1900 would experience vomiting or nausea.

Psychological impact of terminal disease

Much work has examined the prevalence of disease-related symptoms, and several studies have also examined the psychological impact of the disease. Hopwood *et al.* (1991) identified that 27% of women with advanced breast cancer suffered from either anxiety,

Table 2.4   Prevalence of symptoms in patients with cancer and non-cancer

Study	Patients	Pain	Dyspnoea	Fatigue	Vomit	Nausea
Lickiss *et al.* (1994)	mixed ($n = 846$)	60	20	7	–	–
Wilkes (1984)	mixed ($n = 262$)	52	42	–	20	16
Cowley (1993)	mixed ($n = 53$)	66	62	–	–	–
Hockley *et al.* (1988)	mixed ($n = 26$)	69	69	88	27	54
Non-cancer studies						
Cartwright (1991a)	random ($n = 471$)	67	49	–	–	–
Disease-specific studies						
Welch (1991)	HIV ($n = 40$)	–	–	57	–	–
Hicks and Corcoran (1993)	motor neurone disease ($n = 22$)	77	50	–	23	–

depression, or a combination of the two. In a random sample of non-sudden deaths (Wilkes 1984) anxiety was recorded in 24% patients and depression in 18%. This has been supported from other studies of patients with cancer (Coyle *et al.* 1990, Addington Hall *et al.* 1991, Cartwright 1991a, Hardy *et al.* 1994, Hopwood and Stephens 1995) and mixed cancer and non-cancer terminal illness (Cowley 1993, Hicks and Corcoran 1993). Higginson (1995b) estimated that approximately 700 cancer patients and 1600 non-cancer patients per million population per year suffer from acute anxiety fears. In addition, it is recognized that families coping with a terminally ill member may also suffer from psychological distress (Higginson *et al.* 1992b). Using the estimate of one third of families experiencing severe anxiety fears, Higginson (1995b) estimated that 930 families with a terminal cancer patient and 2200 patients with a non-cancer terminally ill relative would suffer. Clearly, palliative care services must address the psychological as well as physical symptoms associated with the disease process, not only in the patient, but also in the family units supporting the patient.

terminal disease (as percentages)

Sleep	Weak	Confused	Loss of appetite	Constipation	Incontinence	Anxiety	Depression
–	35	5		25	–		–
19	52	23	–	–	35	24	18
–	81	38	66	42	51	30	25
88	–	35	–	54	31	–	–
36	38	–	38	32	33	–	36
65	–	–	63	–	–	–	–
64	100	–	–	86	18	32	27

Evidence of need derived from specialist sources

In the UK palliative care services are provided from three main sources: hospital, hospice, and community services. These services contribute different types of care to patients with terminal illness. The hospital services concentrate on symptom control and respite (Hinton 1994b), whereas home care services are chiefly perceived to provide support, symptom management, and counselling (Nash 1993). On average 90% of the last year of a terminally ill patient is spent at home, with home care being highly valued by patients and carers (Neale and Clark 1992).

No figures are available on the precise requirements of the three services, though there is some evidence that patients may not be receiving the care they require. In a needs assessment exercise in Scotland 62% of patients died in hospital compared with 28% at home and 3% in hospices (Scott 1995). Half of these patients preferred to die at home, one quarter in a hospice, and only 10% wished to die in hospital. Only 34% people died in their preferred place of death. People who wished to die at home were unable to do so, owing to poor symptom control. Referrals from general practitioners appear to be frequently related to poor control of symptoms and poor pain management (Seamark *et al.* 1996). Patients who are admitted to hospices generally want the admission, whereas referral to hospitals is only requested by one quarter of patients (Parkes 1985, Bruera *et al.* 1990a). Of cancer patients dying at home 97% felt it was the right place, whereas only half of hospital patients felt the same way (Addington Hall *et al.* 1991). Patients are more likely to die in hospital or hospices if elderly (Cartwright 1993), single, and poor (Komesaroff *et al.* 1989). In general, hospital services have been criticized for poor symptom control, over-treatment, and an uncaring attitude (Wilkes 1984).

Whatever level of provision is offered it is important to stress that most terminal care will continue to be practised in patients' homes and in existing hospitals. The discussion of appropriate levels of hospice provision must not distract from the key role of any hospice, which is to contribute to improvements in the quality of terminal care practised outside its beds. This focal role in education, support and research will only be achieved through close and reciprocal ties between the hospice and existing services. (Frankel and Kammerling 1990)

Current services appear to be geared towards the last few weeks of life, although WHO considers that palliative care should be initiated and developed from diagnosis onwards (Stjernsward *et al.* 1996). There is little evidence of current services adopting this principle. However, in an attempt to overcome this, a palliative care team was established in a hospital service to encourage earlier referral for palliative care (Bennett and Corcoran 1994). Success was gauged by earlier referral within the hospital to this service, with patients being referred to hospice services earlier. Despite the extended duration from referral to death, 80% of patients were still referred within 3 months of their death, and general practitioner referrals to hospice remained short.

In England it has been suggested that 15–25% of cancer deaths receive in-patient hospice care, and 25–65% receive input from a support team or Macmillan nurse (Cartwright 1991a, Addington-Hall *et al.* 1991, Seale 1991b, Higginson 1992b, Higginson 1993a, Bennett and Corcoran 1994). Using these figures, Higginson (1995b) estimated that 700–1800 cancer patients would require support, and 400–700 would require in-patient hospice care per year. For patients with non-cancer progressing illness 350–1400 would require support team and 200–700 would require in-patient palliative care (Higginson 1995b). In the UK, duration of terminal in-patient hospice care varies, though the average is generally between 2 weeks and 1 month prior to death (Rogers *et al.* 1981, James *et al.* 1985, Frankel and Kammerling 1990, Chan and Woodruff 1991, Severs and Wilkins 1991, Cartwright 1993, Rosenthal *et al.* 1993). This closely relates to the recorded deterioration in ability to perform activities of daily living 1 month prior to death (Morris and Sherwood 1987). In the US, the time between application for hospice treatment and death is around 8 weeks (Forster and Lynn 1988). Using the average in-patient duration of stay in the UK and bed occupancy it has been estimated that 40–50 hospice beds are required per million population (Rogers *et al.* 1981, Frankel and Kammerling 1990). However, these figures are likely to be an underestimate of need. Using a wide-ranging consultation process, Nottingham Health identified a number of areas of need, particularly with respect to respite care, pain and symptom control, practical and financial support, and counselling (Nicholas and Frankenburg 1992). In the US unmet needs most frequently revolved around inability to pay medical bills (52%), transport costs (47%), heavy housekeeping (42%), and other activities of daily living (Houts *et al.* 1988, Siegel *et al.* 1992). Need for bereavement services and other emotional burdens on family and friends have also been identified as unmet needs of some services (Neale and Clark 1992, Peace *et al.* 1992, Payne and Relf 1994). In the UK many general practitioners have difficulties in helping relatives and patients cope with emotional stress (Seamark *et al.* 1996).

Needs for specific patient groups

The needs of certain patient groups may be different from those of the majority of patients receiving palliative care. There is a general perception of poor uptake of palliative care services from patients from ethnic minority groups (Hill and Penso 1995), which may be due to failure to appreciate different religious or cultural practices (House 1993). Similarly, hospices which were principally established to meet the need of patients with cancer, have generally failed to provide services for patients with other progressing diseases (Scott 1995, Wilson *et al.* 1995). Diseases which have been highlighted are end stage renal failure (Andrews 1995), heart failure (Beattie 1995), stroke (Wilson *et al.* 1995), and pulmonary diseases (Wilson *et al.* 1995). In areas where referral of non-cancer progressing terminal diseases are encouraged, these may make up one fifth of all referrals (Lickiss *et al.* 1994).

Neurological disease

As Table 2.2 indicates, deaths attributed to neurological disorders are relatively rare, but patients with diseases such as multiple sclerosis and motor neurone disease have different characteristics from patients suffering from cancer, and are likely to require different services from other cancer and non-cancer terminal illness. The key issue for these patients is the long duration of symptoms. Palliative care for these patients revolves around the need for respite care, with only 20% of hospice referrals for terminal care (Hicks and Corcoran 1993).

Patients with HIV and AIDS

There are still relatively few deaths caused by AIDS and related problems, with only 19 deaths per million in men and 2 per million in women in 1995 (Anonymous 1997). In the UK as a whole in 1994, 1189 diagnoses of AIDS were made and there were 1065 deaths from AIDS-related diseases (Higginson 1995b). Despite this relatively small number, the needs of these patients may be quite different from other patients with other terminal illnesses. In general, these patients are considerably younger than most patients receiving palliative care and many may be homeless. AIDS is characterized by acute episodes of infection requiring hospitalization, followed by periods of remission. Mean time from referral to death has been estimated at 31 weeks (Butters *et al.* 1992). Although pain has not been considered a major problem, patients suffering from AIDS experience a multitude of symptoms, particularly related to the pulmonary and gastrointestinal systems and skin problems (Schofferman 1987). The stigma of AIDS, homophobic attitudes, high levels of anxiety caused by lack of effective treatment, and poor symptom control, have all been proposed as reasons for AIDS-specific services (Schofferman 1987), though these are considered uneconomical, and referrals are encouraged to existing hospice services (Higginson 1993a). In one study (Butters *et al.* 1992) 57% of patients suffering from AIDS died in hospital, 22% at home, and 21% in hospices. Others may experience long-term deterioration in health, which will gradually increase the burden on the health services. In the terminal stages of the disease the prevalence of symptoms is frequently higher than for cancer patients. Symptoms are moderate to severe in 35–70% of cases (Cole 1991, Welch 1991, Butters *et al.* 1992).

Childhood diseases

Although there are relatively few children who require palliative care, it must be acknowledged that children's needs may be different from those of adult patients. Deaths due to congenital abnormalities occur most frequently in infants under one year of age (see Table 2.2). Cancer deaths are rarer in this age group, but increase with increasing age. Children's hospices have been developed in Canada (Davies 1996) and children's hospitals provide a specialist service (Goldman *et al.* 1990), but hospices specifically for children have not been advocated in general. For children with terminal illness the aim has been for the child to die at home (Martinson 1980,

Bennett 1984, Chambers 1987, Singleton 1992). Most families of children suffering from cancer take their children home after treatment is stopped, though about a quarter to a third die in hospital (Kohler and Radford 1985, Goldman *et al.* 1990). Clearly, where this is the case, there is a need for the provision of services which can deal with dying children in their own homes.

Conclusions

The palliative care needs of society are likely to change in the future, though the exact magnitude of changes is difficult to gauge accurately. On one hand the incidence of chronic diseases such as cancer appear to be reducing, with more effective treatments on offer. However, this is likely to be counterbalanced by earlier intervention of palliative care services in line with WHO recommendations and further attempts to assess unmet need and intervene where necessary. These unmet needs may be the driving force behind such services in the future.

Question 3

Models of palliative care

CHRIS SALISBURY

What models of palliative care services have been proposed or developed?

This chapter sets out a framework of models of organization for palliative care which have been described in the literature. This framework provides a basis for the evaluation of alternative models which follows in later sections of this book.

In describing models of care, we scrutinized all identified literature which described a functioning or proposed system of organization for the provision of palliative care. This review is limited to models of organization which are specifically concerned with palliative care as opposed to cancer care generally. The framework of options in this section is not necessarily exhaustive. It provides details of models of care which have been described, but many further forms of organization are possible.

The organization of health services in any country is strongly influenced by the financial organization of the healthcare system. The framework described here does not seek to take into account who owns or runs or is responsible for a system, but only how the palliative care service is delivered. Models of care which are superficially similar, such as home care support teams, may in fact be very different in different countries, because of how their role interacts with other services in the system, particularly the provision of community nursing.

In particular it is important to note that the majority of the published studies come from North America, where palliative care has developed in a distinct way for a number of historical and financial reasons (Paradis and Cummings 1986, Kinzbrunner 1994, Taylor 1983). In the UK, palliative care has its roots in the hospice movement which was led by charitable, mainly religious, organizations. From the outset hospices developed an anti-authoritarian, non-institutional model of care (Abel 1986). These initiatives were usually led by doctors, but were multidisciplinary including the central involvement of volunteers. The emphasis was on supporting rather than replacing existing primary care and hospital services.

By contrast, the early North American initiatives in palliative care were led by nurses and volunteers rather than physicians, and emphasized home care rather than in-patient hospices. This was influenced by the Medicare hospice benefit system established in 1982. To be eligible, care must be provided by a multidisciplinary team, primarily at home, and patients must have a primary care-giver (usually a member of their family) (Norwood 1990). The attitude towards other providers was one of competition, as home hospice teams sought to attract 'community dollars' in the 'health industry' (Petersen 1992). Because of differences in the way that palliative care interacts with the rest of the healthcare system in different countries, caution should be used in generalizing from the results of studies in one country to another.

Many organizations identified described themselves as 'hospices', or providing 'hospice care'. As described previously, 'hospice' is a philosophy, rather than a service or a building. It encompasses a range of skills and attitudes which can be delivered through a variety of models of organization. In this review the term 'hospice' will be used when it forms part of an organization's self-description.

Several documents have previously listed the range of alternative models of palliative care, although the frameworks they describe vary according to the date and country in which the review is based (Anonymous 1980, McCabe 1982, Gotay 1983, Saunders and McCorkle 1985, Abel 1986, Anonymous 1990, O'Donnell 1992, SMAC 1992, Higginson 1993a; National Council for Hospice and Specialist Palliative care services 1994, Expert Advisory Group on Cancer 1995, Ford 1995, Higginson 1995b, Hospice Information Service 1996, Taylor 1983). A useful series of papers published in 1990–92 describes the provision of palliative care in a range of developed countries (Albrecht 1990, Lichter 1990, Gomez-Baptiste 1992, Magno 1992). Most reviews categorize models of care within a general framework of in-patient services in hospitals, free-standing hospices, day care, and home care teams.

These categories however are not clearly defined or mutually exclusive, and include organizations which are highly variable. Some provide one of the above services, and others integrate several forms of care. There are further approaches to palliative care which do not fall neatly into any of these categories.

A comprehensive framework of alternative models of palliative care is described below. References to papers which describe each approach can be found below and in Table 3.1. Not all articles which were reviewed are referenced here or detailed in the table, as many papers provided very limited information. The table gives examples of descriptive studies of the various models.

Hospital approaches

Consultation teams

Hospital palliative care support teams were pioneered in the UK at St Thomas's Hospital in the late 1970s (Bates *et al.* 1981). They are variously described under the terms 'support teams', 'palliative care teams', symptom control teams', or under the umbrella term 'hospice' in the US. They bring the principles and benefits of palliative care into acute hospitals. These teams are multidisciplinary, normally including doctors, nurses, social workers, and often a chaplain and other staff. They provide an advisory service to the team with primary responsibility for the patient in hospital, rather than having dedicated beds of their own. Such teams have been described in a number of countries including the UK (Bates *et al.* 1981, Herxheimer *et al.* 1985, Hockley *et al.* 1988, Hockley 1990, Simpson 1991, Ellershaw *et al.* 1995, Hockley 1996, McQuillan *et al.* 1996), Canada (Mount 1980, Bruera 1989), and Australia (Kramer and Dwyer 1989, Lickiss *et al.* 1994), but most of the literature comes from the US (Winstead *et al.* 1980, Richardson *et al.* 1987, Carlson *et al.* 1988, Woodruff *et al.* 1991, Weissman and Griffie 1994). The institution of palliative care teams in hospital is not always problem free because of issues of staffing, clinical responsibility, leadership, and communication (Herxheimer *et al.* 1985).

The aims of hospital support teams include providing assistance in the relief of symptoms, emotional social and spiritual support to patients, counselling and support to the bereaved, help with placement, advice to staff, and educational and research programmes. The multidisciplinary composition of teams varies according to local needs and resources. As Hockey (1992) notes,

Table 3.1   UK studies of palliative home care nurses – examples of

Author	Country	Years(s)	Setting	Disease
Weller (1981)	UK	1978–80	home care team	Cancer
Pettingale (1986)	UK	1982–85	hospice at home/ specialist outreach	Mixed
Clench (1986)	UK	Not applicable	home care team	Mixed
Walton (1987)	UK	Not applicable	Not applicable	Mixed
Ward (1987)	UK	1984	home care team, hospice	Mixed
Lunt and Yardley (1988)	UK	1985	home care team	Mixed
Doyle (1991)	UK	1977–87	home care team	Cancer
Addington Hall *et al.* (1992)	UK	1987–90	All settings	Cancer
Ford (1992)	UK	Not applicable	home care team, hospice	Cancer
Bergen (1992)	UK	Not known	family unit	Mixed
Higginson *et al.* (1992b)	UK	Not known	home care team	Cancer
(Hockey 1994)	UK	1988–89	home care team	Mixed
Boyd (1995)	UK	1992	home care team	Mixed
Chambers and Oakhill (1995)	UK	Not applicable	All settings	Cancer
Robbins *et al.* (1997)	UK	1995–96	home care team	Mixed

descriptions or evaluations

Study	Brief key points
description of process of care (no detailed data)	Personal and subjective description of delivery of home care to cancer patients by one nurse
observational study (detailed data)	Description of operation and workload of Camberwell terminal care support team
description of process of care (no detailed data)	Description of functioning of Dorothy House Foundation, a community based domiciliary support service and limited data about activity. Discussion of advantages of community based model
authoritative opinion	Describes potential merits of Macmillan nurses in advising about home care for dying patients
Observational study (detailed data)	Studies of 8 home care services, 4 attached to hospital, 4 home care only. 65% of patients of latter died at home, cf. 29% of patients at hospital attached services. Wide variation in staffing and organization between home care services
Interview survey, questionnaire survey	Description of work of specialist Macmillan nurses in terminal care. Detailed report of activity based on interviews, questionnaire and diary study. See also Lunt and Neale (1987).
Retrospective study	Description of 10 yrs cases dealt with by St Columbus Home Care Service. A hospice based multidisciplinary team. See also Doyle (1980). Descriptive paper, no attempt to evaluate service
Interview survey, RCT	Evaluation of nurses who co-ordinated NHS, voluntary, and local authority services
authoritative opinion	Review of growth of Marie Curie organization. Provides (1) 11 inpt centres; (2) 5000 'hands on' nurses providing day, night, and respite care; (3) education dept
interview survey	Case studies of 36 district nurses and 2 Macmillan nurses. Nurses' views about patients' needs and extent to which standards of care were achieved
Observational study (detailed data)	Description of community based support teams with detailed data. Validation of Support Team Assessment Schedule
interview survey, retrospective study	Description of work of home care service of one hospice, and brief evaluation of the extent to which it meets its aims.
questionnaire survey	In survey of general practitioners, most approved of palliative home care team. Wanted them to extend their service to share out of hours cover. As most general practitioners now using deputies or cooperatives the role of specialist team at night is at least as important out-of-hours as it is in the day
description of process of care (no detailed data)	Use of paediatric oncology nurses to link primary healthcare team, regional hospital, and tertiary referral centre
questionnaire survey	Evaluation of home nursing service through views of general practitioners, nurses and bereaved nurses

little research has been done about the best team size in relation to case-load.

In some hospitals advice comes from individual palliative care nurse specialists, or from palliative care consultants, who do not necessarily have the support of a multidisciplinary team. An example of the work of a nurse specialist is described in the SUPPORT study from the US (Connors *et al.* 1995). A growing trend is for specialist palliative care nurses who provide advice, support, and co-ordination of services for patients with specific diseases.

Specialist palliative care ward in hospital

A separate unit for terminal care in a general hospital was developed as a model in Canada, but has been described in a number of countries (Mount 1980, Wilson *et al.* 1983, Greer *et al.* 1986, Hoskin and Hanks 1988, Barrelet and Jousson 1993, Kellar *et al.* 1996). The best known example of this model is the unit in Montreal's Royal Victoria Hospital (Mount 1980). This model is less common in the UK, where special units have generally developed apart from existing hospitals, but a special unit for the terminally ill elderly has been described in Portsmouth (Severs and Wilkins 1991). The claimed advantages and disadvantages of siting palliative care units within or separately from hospitals have been described (Mount 1980, Gotay 1983).

Encouraging a palliative care approach amongst non-specialist staff

Hospital palliative care support teams usually include the education of nursing and medical staff throughout the hospital as one of their aims, offering teaching about the palliative care approach. One of the claimed advantages of the hospital support team, which advises about in-patients but does not take over primary clinical responsibility, is that good practice is widely disseminated (Bates *et al.* 1981, McQuillan *et al.* 1996). However, an alternative model of care is to aim to deliver high quality palliative care for all patients by making the education of non-specialist staff the main priority. This was indeed one of the main recommendations of the Wilkes report (1980). The use of a hospital-wide educational initiative has been described (Zorzitto *et al.* 1989). Similarly the use of guidelines to encourage consistently high standards of palliative care in the community has been described (Robinson and Stacy 1994).

Free-standing hospices

Although, as discussed, the term 'hospice' refers to an approach rather than a building or facility, it has through common usage also been applied to free-standing units providing palliative care. These units may or may not provide in-patient care, day care, home care, advisory services, bereavement services, and other services.

In-patient services in free-standing units in the UK were originally supported by voluntary, charitable organizations (Marie Curie, Sue Ryder, and others), but more latterly some were instituted by the NHS. The philosophy of care builds on that established at St Christopher's hospice, and is quite distinct from that of hospitals. It involves a personal non-institutional, approach, promoting psychological and physical well-being though good symptom control. The whole-person approach respects patient's autonomy and choices, and open communication is encouraged. All units have multidisciplinary staff, and many rely heavily on volunteer help. Although these free-standing hospices are common in the UK, detailed descriptions of their activities are relatively few, with several coming from one hospice, St Christopher's (Parkes 1979, Burne 1984, Manning 1984, Parkes and Parkes 1984, Parkes 1985, Dominica 1987, Ford 1992).

Institutional services for patients who are not in-patients

Out-patient clinics

Most palliative care consultants provide out-patient consultation services at their hospital or hospice base, although only limited description and no evaluations of this service were identified (Parkes 1980).

Day care

Day care may be provided by specialist palliative care teams, as an adjunct to in-patient facilities or in free-standing centres without in-patient beds. These units provide rehabilitation and social activities, respite for carers, and in some cases patients can see the doctor for review of treatment (Clench 1986, Doyle 1991, Faulkner *et al.* 1993). Although the 1980 Standing Medical Advisory Committee (Wilkes 1980) recommended that the advantages of day care should be carefully examined, descriptions and evaluations of this model of care remain very sparse.

Home-based services

Family

It should not be forgotten that for most patients dying at home, the major burden of care falls on the patient's family. Several authors have described the important contribution made by families (Reilly and Patten 1981, Haines and Booroff 1986, Aldridge 1987, Martens and Davies 1990).

Primary healthcare team

In the UK the family are supported by community nurses and general practitioners within the primary healthcare team. Several authors have described the contribution to care which can be made by the primary healthcare team, who have often known the patient long before the terminal illness, and will continue to care for the family afterwards (Haines and Booroff 1986, Aldridge 1987, Mabbott and Rothery 1988, Gomas 1993, Wakefield *et al.* 1993, Robinson and Stacy 1994). The primary healthcare team may also care for people in residential nursing homes rather than their own homes (Cartwright 1991c).

Hospice home care nurse

The patient, family, and primary healthcare team are in turn supported by an array of home care nurses. This model of care is highly variable. Nurses may provide advice or hands-on nursing care, they may work in a nursing team or within a multidisciplinary home care support team, they may be based in a free-standing hospice, a hospital, or independently, and their functions may vary, particularly between countries according to the healthcare system. Details of references are shown in Table 3.1. This table is limited to studies from the UK, as the work of home care nurses is not comparable in other health systems.

Specialist nurses in the UK were mainly originally funded by the Cancer Relief Macmillan Fund and known as 'Macmillan nurses'. Their role is to provide advice about symptom control and pain relief and emotional support to the patient and his/her family, and to act as a resource and liaison with the specialist palliative care services. Macmillan nurses do not take over responsibility from district nurses for practical nursing. As district nurses take an increasing role in planning care for their patients, delegating practical tasks to nursing assistants, the interface between the district nurse and the Macmillan nurse has in some areas become unclear.

Marie Curie nurses provide a night nursing service, including 'hands-on' practical nursing, which complements the daytime community nursing service.

Multidisciplinary home care support team

The home care nurses previously described may work as part of a multidisciplinary team, including doctors, social workers, and others. Such a team may be based in hospital (Hockley 1996), hospice (Parkes 1980, Doyle 1991), or community (Clench 1986). It can provide wide-ranging advice to general practitioners and district nurses, including telephone advice, domiciliary consultations, and arranging respite day care or in-patient admission when necessary (Doyle 1980, Parkes 1980, Doyle 1991, Higginson *et al.* 1992b). The concept of a home support team therefore encompasses a wide range of forms of organization with different roles (Higginson 1993a). Teams have been described and proposed which cater specifically for terminally ill children (Chambers *et al.* 1989, Levy *et al.* 1990), or for terminal care in AIDS (Smits *et al.* 1990, Butters *et al.* 1992).

One important issue for home care support teams is the provision of care outside normal working hours. In the UK, general practitioners have expressed a need for expansion in palliative care support to include evenings and weekends (Boyd 1995). In countries without universal primary care, this issue is of even greater importance, as a lack of home support during unsocial hours is a frequent cause of hospital admission (Beck Friis and Strang 1993a, Gardner Nix *et al.* 1995). This has influenced the development of home care teams providing 24 hour care.

In a number of countries home care teams have been described which have a different range of functions from those operating in the UK. In North America, for example, the home care advisory team may focus on making arrangements for patients discharged from hospital and co-ordinating hospital services for patients based at home (Ophof *et al.* 1989, Singleton 1992). In the US and in Italy, home care teams act more as providers of care than advisors (Hadlock 1985, Ventafridda *et al.* 1989, Mercadante *et al.* 1992). This is related to the less developed system of primary healthcare in these countries. In Canada a network of six general practitioners have developed a palliative care support service to provide care across the city of Scarborough, by providing advice to the patient's own general practitioner (Gardner Nix *et al.* 1995).

Many of the studies of home-based palliative care come from the US (Barzelai 1981, Silver 1981, Wilson *et al.* 1983, Kane *et al.* 1984, Zimmer *et al.* 1984, Zimmer *et al.* 1985, Greer *et al.* 1986, Greer and Mor 1986, Petersen 1992), where this model is common as a result of the Medicare reimbursement requirements previously described. It is unclear how far the American experience is relevant to the UK.

Comprehensive hospital at home

Patients requiring intensive nursing care are normally admitted to a hospital or in-patient hospice unit. Several countries have experimented with the model of providing comprehensive nursing services at home, including in some cases interventionizt procedures such as intravenous lines and blood transfusions. The use of this model of 'hospital at home' has been described for a variety of diseases, and a number of descriptions of services specifically describe terminal care (Anand *et al.* 1989, Pannuti and Tanneberger 1992, Beck Friis and Strang 1993a). The longest running example of this service in the UK is described in Peterborough (Anand *et al.* 1989). The original concept of a 'hospital outreach' programme has evolved into a service which is integrated with existing community nursing and general practitioner services. Patients are cared for with a range of conditions, but terminally ill patients account for 40% of the case-load. More recently the development of a hospice at home service for patients with HIV/AIDS has been described (Koffman *et al.* 1996).

Other services

One interesting model of care is the use of group support, whereby concepts of group work developed in psychiatry are used to improve coping strategies in terminally ill patients. A well-conducted randomized prospective outcome study showed that this concept resulted in significant psychological benefits for patients (Spiegel *et al.* 1981).

The work of volunteers is an important component of many hospice services, although their contribution has rarely been described, except in passing. The use of volunteers in a structured way as a supportive friend or 'buddy' was developed in the US in the context of caring for patients with AIDS. Within the UK, voluntary and self-help organizations have also been particularly active in the field of HIV (Anonymous 1989, Partridge 1989, Singh 1989, Thomson 1989). An adaptation of this model to provide help for patients with a range of terminal illnesses has been described in Australia (McCallum *et al.* 1989).

An intriguing study from the US examined the use of an automated system to maintain contact with patients dying at home (Siegel *et al.* 1992). A computer telephoned the patients at regular intervals and asked them to leave a message if they had any unmet needs or needed help from a social worker. The group of patients in the trial had fewer unmet needs, although the conclusions were not statistically significant owing to the small number of patients studied. Whether such an impersonal system would attract support in other countries is debatable.

Integrated services providing several forms of care

The above framework describes various ways of providing palliative care. Some services aim to meet one aspect of the patients overall needs (e.g. group support for psychological needs) other services provide fairly global care and advice (hospice home care nurses, general practitioners). Different models of care may not necessarily be alternatives, as they may each have contributions for different purposes, or for patients at different stages of the disease process. Specialist palliative care services have been developed in several countries, which provide several of the above services in an integrated way (Mount 1980, Winstead *et al.* 1980, Bates *et al.*

1981, Turnbull 1981, Dominica 1987, Fothergill Bourbonnais 1988, Maddocks 1990, Walsh 1990, Lickiss *et al.* 1994, Maddocks *et al.* 1994, Hockley 1996, Lovel 1996). British palliative care teams commonly provide in-patient beds, respite care, day care, domiciliary home care nurses, bereavement care, education, and research programmes (Parkes 1985, Oliver 1996).

To some extent the models which are described in the literature represent options for healthcare planners (Clark *et al.* 1995a, Ford 1995). A useful recent review from the US highlighted the importance of a sound research base to support effective policy decisions (Anonymous 1996a). However, evidence that one model of care is more effective than another in one setting does not mean that another model of care is not also valuable, and possibly more valuable, in another setting. Such choices, if evidence-based, will require comparisons between alternative models of palliative care, and cost utility assessment. In fact the majority of the literature is comprised of simple descriptions of the process of care. Few studies involve comparisons between alternative models, and those comparative studies which have been done have mainly compared one form of palliative care with 'conventional care'. There has been little attempt to relate different models of organization to anticipated improved outcomes (Johnston and Abraham 1995). Later chapters of this book seek to summarize the findings of the available research about the impact on defined outcomes such as patient satisfaction and quality of life.

Question 4 ....
Costs and benefits

NICK BOSANQUET

What evidence is available about the costs and benefits of various models of palliative care?

Starting from a common inspiration in the hospice movement, palliative care in the US and the UK has shown very different patterns of development reacting to different local incentives. This difference in development has also affected the types of evaluation carried out. In many respects the US has taken the lead with a more impressive body of evidence on multi-unit studies of costs and effectiveness. The hospice movement in the US has had to fight hard for funds and this critical scrutiny has generated activity in trials. For the UK the main focus has been on the collection of evidence to improve patient care within units. There is little evidence from the UK either on comparative costs or on the comparative effectiveness of different methods of care, for example hospice as against home-based care.

Evidence from North America

The key study in the US is still the National Hospice Study (Greer *et al*. 1986). Mount and Scott (1983) had provided an earlier discussion of some of the problems in methodology before the results were known. This covered 833 home-care-based patients, 624 hospital-based hospice patients, and 297 patients in conventional care. The study was carried out in 1981–83 and compared results on a variety of outcome measures for quality of life, social functioning, pain control, and carer satisfaction.

Despite the substantial variation in the pattern of care we were unable to detect significant differences in patient quality of life attributable to hospice with the possible exception of pain control. (Greer *et al*. 1986)

Hospice care was certainly no worse than conventional care but it did not seem to lead to much better outcomes for patients either in clinical or social terms.

Careful analysis of the interrelationship between patients' receipt of intensive services, physician specialty, and the assessed aggressiveness of the physician reveals that hospice–nonhospice is the dominant effect. Patients and families may choose settings that reflect their values and desire for palliative care, and physicians, regardless of specialty, may choose to practice in or in conjunction with such settings. If this perspective is true, the treatment differences may be largely attributable to selection bias. Alternately, since home care patients are more likely to be home where medical procedures are generally not performed, their use rate would obviously be lower than those of conventional care patients. Additionally, observations of many of the hospital based hospices, both demonstration and nondemonstration, point to the pervasiveness of the palliative philosophy, apparently influencing even the behaviour of nonhospice physicians. (Greer *et al.* 1986)

For costs there were some clear differences between home care and other forms of care. Home care had costs which were considerably less than those of hospital or conventional care, but the costs of hospital-based hospice care were the same as those of conventional care except in the last month of life. With home care most of the reduction in costs resulted from a larger contribution of informal care 'relying on family members to provide up to 12 hours a day of direct care'. The Study warned that hospice costs might rise in the future with longer stays and greater severity of illness. It concluded that 'despite these concerns about future cost trends, the NHS appears to confirm that hospice is a viable alternative for the care of some terminal patients. Such alternatives are justifiable in a pluralistic society'.

The National Hospice Study has been criticized for lack of randomization. The critique is summarized in Aitken (1986), but its results were substantially confirmed in one of the few randomized controlled trials ever to be carried out on palliative care, that by Kane *et al.* (1984). In this study patients were allocated randomly between hospice care and conventional care in a teaching hospital. There were no differences in pain, symptom relief, or alleviation of psychological distress from hospice care: however, patients and their families showed higher satisfaction with hospice care. There were no significant differences in cost per case. A critique of this study is found in Mahoney (1986). Torrens (1985) draws lessons from these early studies and criticizes the lack of rational and appropriate distribution of the service:

We can no longer assume that if one hospice programme is good, 1400 are better. Nor can we assume that the current 1400 hospice places are necessarily in the right places, delivering the right services, and effectively serving the exact populations they should.

Buckingham and Lupu (1982) had also shown the wide variety of hospices offering different services with very different costs. The most extreme criticism of hospices are to be found in Gibson (1984):

The potential negative consequences of the hospice program are numerous and serious. There is no clear economic necessity for embarking on such a morally dangerous path, yet the nation has already gone a considerable distance in this direction.

Later studies have substantially confirmed these earlier mixed results, although often with a more positive interpretation of the costs and benefits of home care. Zimmer *et al.* (1985) carried out a randomized trial of home care showing higher carer satisfaction and lower costs. Thus Hughes *et al.* (1992) compared a hospital-based home care team with conventional care. There were no differences in patient survival, activities of daily living, cognitive functioning, or morale, but significant increases in patient and care-giver satisfaction. Health service use was also lower in the home care groups so that their costs were lower. A survey by Emanuel (1996) concludes that hospice and advance directives can save between 25% and 40% of healthcare costs during the last months of life with decreasing savings over longer periods:

... the savings from hospice are predominantly the result of the reduced use of hospital care (Medicare Part A expenditures) in the last month of life. Medicare patients receiving hospice had a savings of $6601 in nonhospice Part A and $950 in Part B Medicare payments over the last 12 months of their lives. This means that more than 85% of the savings are from Part A expenditures—payments for in-patient services. However, most of the savings are in the last month of life, in which hospice patients had a savings of $5231 in nonhospice Part A and $862 in Part B Medicare payments. Reduced use of hospitals in the last month of life, therefore, accounts for almost 70% of savings from hospice in the last year of life. Other studies of hospice also demonstrate significant reductions in hospital use concentrated in the last month of life. This indicates that most of the savings from hospice is a result of reduced use of in-patient services during the last month of life. (Emanuel 1996)

A local study in Greenville, South Carolina showed gains in the last 3 months. This study was not randomized but of two groups comparable in diagnoses, sex, race, payer status, and age (Mitchell *et al.* 1994). The earlier studies in the 1980s seemed to have shifted the direction of development towards home care by special teams. Evaluation in paediatric care had already shown very positive results in reducing the cost of care (Moldow *et al.* 1982). A later study, however, showed that home care could substantially raise the in-direct and out-of-pocket costs incurred by families (Schweitzer *et al.* 1993). As Kane (1986) had pointed out in drawing lessons from hospice evaluations:

Ironically, were the hospice advocates to abandon some of their more extravagant claims, there would be no controversy about the role of the hospice as a legitimate form of therapy.

A meta-analysis of whether educational and psychosocial care helped adults with cancer showed statistically significant and beneficial effects for all seven chosen outcomes—anxiety, depression, mood, nausea, vomiting, pain, and knowledge (Devine and Westlake 1995). The authors conclude that the results are strong and well based. Pawling Kaplan and O'Connor (1989) also report positive results for a palliative care team in an inner city area.

Concern about costs of ineffective therapies in the last year of life have increased sympathy for the hospice approach. A study of the results of intensive care for critically ill cancer patients showed very poor results with many dying in the unit and 70–80% dying within 3 months even if discharged.

Attempts to save these patients incur considerable costs that may affect the families of these patients. The findings outlined in this study regarding survival, meaningful survival and the cost to achieve these outcomes should encourage physicians to discuss these topics with patients and their families. (Schapira *et al.* 1993)

However, the most comprehensive review of cost-saving measures (Emanuel and Emanuel 1994) concluded that reducing such inter-ventions would save at most 3.3% of total health expenditures. Nevertheless, there were substantial arguments for such measures as hospice care in any case: `

Respecting patients' wishes, reducing pain and suffering and providing compassionate and dignified care at the end of life have overwhelming merit.

Evidence from the UK

Evaluation studies in the UK made promising beginnings with early evaluations of St Christopher's Hospice by Parkes (1979, 1980) and a study by Hinton (1979). These showed that hospice care could be more effective than hospital care, although the numbers involved in the studies were small. For the next two decades most studies were descriptive. A good case study of a single service was that of Hockey (1994). This brought together data from a range of sources including general practitioners, patients, carers, and hospital staff to record views, contacts, and activities. In general satisfaction was high but there seemed to be a need for better collaboration between community staff and the specialist services.

The difficulties of setting up evaluations were well discussed by Goddard (1993) and by Higginson and McCarthy (1989) who also provided a critique of US studies. In the mid-1990s some studies began to appear. Ellershaw *et al.* (1995) assessed the effectiveness of a hospital based team, and Raftery *et al.* (1996) carried out an randomized controlled trial of a district co-ordinating service for patients with terminal illness.

The objective of this paper is to compare the cost-effectiveness of a co-ordination service with standard services for terminally ill cancer patients with a prognosis of less than one year.

We designed a randomized controlled trial, with patients randomized by the general practice with which they were registered. Co-ordination group patients received the assistance of two nurse coordinators whose role was to ensure that patients had access to appropriate services.

The setting was in a South London health authority. Complete service use and outcome data were collected on 167 patients, 86 in the co-ordination group, and 81 in the control group.

Our results as previously reported, show that no differences in outcomes were detected between the co-ordination and control groups; the mean total costs incurred by the co-ordination group were significantly less than those of the control group. The co-ordinated group used significantly fewer in-patient days (mean 24 versus 40 in-patient days; $t = 2.4$, $p = 0.002$) and nurse home visits (mean 14.5 versus 37.5 visits; $t = 0.3$, $p = 0.01$). Mean cost per co-ordinated patient was almost half that of the control group patients (£4774 versus £8034, $t = 2.8$, $p = 0.006$). Although the unit cost data were relatively crude, these cost reductions were insensitive to a wide range of unit costs. These differences persisted when, in order to control for any putative differences in severity between the two groups, the analysis was restricted to patients who had died by the end of the study. The ratio of potential cost savings to the cost of co-ordination service was between 4 : 1 and 8 : 1.

In conclusion, the co-ordination service for cancer patients who were terminally ill with a prognosis of less than one year was more cost effective than standard services, due to achieving the same outcomes at lower service use, particularly in-patient days in acute hospital. Assuming that the observed effects are real, improved co-ordination of palliative care offers the potential for considerable savings. Further research is needed to explore the issue. (Raftery *et al.* 1996)

Co-ordination group patients received the assistance of two nurse co-ordinators whose role was to ensure that patients had access to appropriate services. The co-ordinated group used significantly fewer in-patient day and nurse home visits. Mean cost per co-ordinated patient was almost half that of the control group patients (£4774 versus £8034).

Most development in the UK was concerned with quality assurance—mainly in terms of help to individual units to provide improved process. Ingleton and Faulkner (1995a) provide a good review of the range of possible methods and of the literature (Ingleton and Faulkner 1995b). Higginson (1994) surveys methods of clinical and organizational audit. Higginson *et al.* (1992b) report on instruments which can help support teams to improve their performance, and Neale *et al.* (1993) provide a review of the literature on purchasing palliative care.

The UK literature on costs is sparse. Tierney *et al.* (1994) provide a summary of the methodology. An early survey of costs covering 40 hospices is that of Hill and Oliver (1988). This showed a range of costs ranging from £373 to £559 per patient week. Costs per week seemed to fall with size of hospice. This was a useful study but it has not been followed up. Within the UK there has been most activity in comparing units in costs and activities in Scotland. Kindlen (1988) provides data on a postal survey of the activities of home care services. Sims (1995) shows shifts in income sources from voluntary donation to health board grants in the course of the 1990s, and King *et al.* (1993) review different accounting systems used by palliative care in Scotland. Most of these later studies were stimulated by the problems of contracting in the internal market.

The substantial commitment made to hospices and palliative care over the previous two decades was made without any hard information on either comparative costs or comparative benefits. The absence of information is particularly striking on capital costs and on the relative costs of benefits of home care as against hospice in-patient service. Thus very substantial investment (more than £500 m over the last decade) and current revenue spending of £300–500 m a year has been committed without any information about relative costs or effectiveness.

Evidence from outside the US and the UK

Outside the US and the UK the literature is sparse. Gray *et al.* (1987) made a pioneering attempt to compare the cost of home-based and hospital care in Western Australia. For matched groups there were no savings from home-based care:

This study has shown that it can take as much time and professional effort to provide terminal care in the home as to continue to pursue treatment in hospital.

Also in Australia, Glare and Lickiss (1992) set out some interesting approaches to quality assurance involving team discussions of bad outcomes including uncontrolled symptoms for more than 24 hours, death without dignity, unscheduled admissions, and dissatisfied patients

In Canada, Jarvis *et al.* (1996) carried out a study of a large regional and tertiary care facility. Outcomes covered included quality of life, satisfaction for carers, and good morale and low stress for staff.

Italy has been exceptional in supplying a number of studies showing positive outcomes and reduced costs from home care for cancer patients (Ventafridda *et al.* 1989, Mercadante *et al.* 1992, Pannuti and Tanneberger 1992) and for patients with AIDS (Anonymous 1982). These studies were mostly on a small scale and over short time periods, but they showed very considerable savings—in one case a cost of L 52 500 (£19) for a day's home care, compared to L 360 000 (£132) for a day's hospitalization.

The data which emerged have shown that home care produced results equivalent to those achieved in hospital, as far as clinical parameters are concerned, showing, at the same time, better results as far as psychological and social parameters are concerned in the home care group.

It is therefore important to note how the care environment which can be achieved in the patient's home is anything but a limitation of therapeutic possibilities. Pain and other symptoms can be controlled by the use of an appropriate pharmacological strategy in the home too. In fact, the WHO sequential scale has showed itself able to control pain, with a reduction of about ⅔ in the home care group and ½ in the hospitalized one, without requiring complicated care structures. From this point of view the choice of administering analgesics at previously established times, rather than when needed, is certainly an important element. This administration schedule allows the patient and family greater independence, and helps to forestall accentuation of the pain situation, instead of resorting to emergency treatment when pain occurs. In psychological terms, this approach helps the immediate family to live more calmly since a real control, in preventive terms, is experienced and expectations of the pain experience are reduced.

In the same way, it should be observed that the degree of autonomy or movement which patients are able to achieve is higher in the home environment than in hospital after two weeks' treatment. . . . After 14 days, patients at home appear to be more active. It is thus legitimate to suppose that such a difference is due not so much to the extra freedom of movement at home as to the higher stimulation conditions which favour some recovery of patients autonomy and activity. This more intense recovery, although limited by the advanced conditions of the illness, has a profound psychological impact, since it constitutes a strength and an impulse to recover a healthier image of oneself, including aspects of one's own autonomy and independence.

Another important data, summarized in an overall value, is the quality of life index which, at T 14, is better in patients cared for at home. The total value consists of the sum of the scores in single areas, concerning support received, mood, degree of health, degree of activity, and daily life. The fact that differences are detectable between home and the hospital therefore leads to the conclusion that the two approaches to care cannot only be distinguished by the place in which treatment takes place, but also by their effect on the mood of and support received by the patient.

In other words, it can be said that being cared for at home or in hospital does not so much affect pain control (similar in both environments), as other dimensions, which are more qualitative and related to the patient's experience of his situation. (Ventafridda *et al.* 1989)

Conclusions

Early studies concentrate on whether hospice care should exist at all: now the issues are more limited to collection of evidence on particular types of services. There is a considerable body of international evidence showing the effectiveness of low cost, home based interventions (Table 4.1). Randomized controlled trials may well continue to be virtually impossible, but the way seems clear for much more research at a local level to give practical help in decisions about service organization and communication with patients and carers.

Table 4.1 Comparative studies on costs and benefits of various models of palliative care

Authors country	Study design	Comparison	Outcome	Results (key conclusions)
Kane *et al.* (1984) USA	Randomized controlled trial	Hospice *vs* hospital treatment	Costs Quality of life and symptoms Satisfaction	Hospice $11 618; controls $11 614 No significant differences in pain control, symptom scores, activities of daily living but there were in satisfaction scores Hospices did not yield expected benefits but high level of satisfaction
Zimmer *et al.* (1985) USA	Randomized controlled trial	Home care team vs. controls	Costs Satisfaction Quality of life Service utilization	Hospital team $22.27, control $36.44 Carer satisfaction 99.8 team, 88.8 control Functional ability not greater but carers more satisfied Intervention was to lower costs—fewer hospitalizations/nursing home admissions and up visits
Ventafridda *et al.* (1989) Italy	Observational study	Hospital v home care	Costs Quality of life Satisfaction	Costs L52 500/day home care, L360 000/day hospital On Spitzer health Scale 56% of hospital patients felt very ill; in home care sample 23% did. For total index better average value in home care Results seen as better for home care in 'psychological' and 'social' parameters *Home care presented as very positive*
Hughes *et al.* (1992) USA	Randomized controlled trial	Home care team vs. conventional care	Costs Functional status and psychological status Satisfaction	Costs 18% lower in home care group No differences in ADL on cognitive functioning Significant increase in in-patient and care-giver satisfaction. *Intervention seen as highly positive*
Raftery *et al.* (1996) UK	Randomized controlled trial	Nurse co-ordinators attached to practices vs. controls	Costs Symptom control and quality of life Depression and anxiety Use of services	Co-ordinator group had 24 vs 40 in-patient days and nurse home visits : mean cost £4774 per patient co-ordinators v £8034 control Outcomes—symptom control/quality of care did not differ between the 2 groups positive *Co-ordination at practice level seen as effective*

Question 5 ....

Contemporary models for palliative care nursing

MARIA LORENTZON

What is the appropriate skill-mix in palliative care nursing in terms of specialist and general nursing skills? What are the costs and benefits associated with the clinical nurse specialist role in palliative care?

Palliative care has expanded rapidly as a specialist healthcare discipline during the past few decades, especially in North America, as will be evident in the literature review which follows. Development of this area of healthcare has also been evident in the UK, and the role of Cecily Saunders is notable in this context. The multi-disciplinary approach which typifies this field of healthcare is encapsulated in her person, being qualified as a nurse, doctor, and social worker. Nursing input to caring for the dying has been prominent for several hundred years. In medieval times care of the body was overshadowed by concern for the souls of dying patients. Following the Reformation and dissolution of the monasteries a more secular approach prevailed in the hospitals of Protestant countries such as Britain. This is exemplified in the eighteenth and nineteenth century British hospital foundations which were initiated and supported by wealthy benefactors. The spiritual motivation was not absent in these hospitals, although their administration was not in the hands of religious authorities. Care of the dying has, not surprisingly, attracted many individuals with religious belief and several facilities for palliative care are in the hands of monastic and other Christian organizations.

Involvement by nurses in the holistic care of dying patients has been extensive. The tendency to regard death as 'medical failure' may have inhibited major participation by doctors in palliative care until comparatively recently. Medieval doctors withdrew completely from treating dying patients, leaving the role of ministering to patients to priests. The reason was mainly that it would be viewed as dishonest to collect a doctor's fee if no cure seemed possible. More active participation in palliative care by doctors in the UK was signalled through the recognition of the specialist in palliative medicine by the Royal College of Physicians in 1987. This increased involvement by medical practitioners enhanced the multi-disciplinary ethos in palliative care, especially in the area of symptom relief.

Acknowledging the increasing demands on palliative care services, expanding beyond the traditional concentration on cancer and, more recently, on AIDS to other disease categories, the UK Department of Health has recognized the need to ensure that comprehensive and cost-effective palliative care services are being offered within the NHS. In view of the specific interest in cost-effectiveness of services, it is significant that the nursing literature reviewed in this project presented virtually no direct information on costs as will be discussed in this chapter.

The context in which the review was conducted took account of the following factors which have been highlighted in a previous chapter:

- the increased importance of the NHS as funder of palliative care services
- the need to develop new partnerships between specialist and informal service providers in palliative care
- the need to adjust palliative care services to the changing organizational pattern of the NHS
- the increasing complexity of palliative care services
- the increasing emphasis on community based care and on the role of informal carers
- the increasing concern about effectiveness and value for money in the currently available palliative care services.

The last-mentioned point forms the main focus for this chapter.

Methodology

Initial examination of available publications revealed virtually no information on costs in relation to benefits of nursing services. Furthermore, 'skill-mix' was not specifically addressed and therefore 'role' was examined as a substitute, in order to piece together the desirable components thought to encompass 'the palliative care nurse'. Specialist and advanced practice were considered jointly with no attempt to distinguish between them.

A total of 103 documents were identified as relevant to the research question. However, many of these papers described small-scale studies, using unrepresentative samples. This reduced the power of the data in terms of ability to generalize from conclusions drawn by researchers. Most of the nursing research was descriptive rather than experimental, adopting a qualitative research methodology. Many themes other than those related to the specific question emerged; for example, staff stress and provision of psychological/emotional support for patients and relatives. These were briefly considered, although the main emphasis was placed on the components of the research question. The review therefore included both qualitative and quantitative research with wide variety of outcome measures. The review revealed very few studies using an experimental design and hardly any issues were addressed in more than one comparable, experimental study.

Discussion in this chapter will centre on the following themes:

- general nursing roles (including individual and team-based functions)
- nursing roles in hospices
- nursing roles in hospitals and in the community
- specialist and advanced nursing practice
- psychological support of patients and stress among nurses.

General nursing roles

Individual roles

An excellent summary of the key areas in terminal care nursing is provided in the opening chapter of *Nursing issues and research in terminal care* by Wilson-Barnett and Raiman (1988a). In this account of the main aspects of nursing the dying Wilson-Barnett draws on many relevant sources. Her introductory sentence forms a fitting opening to our discussion about the general role of the palliative care nurse. She says: 'Caring for the dying person and his family extends all the fundamental skills a nurse should have.' Examination of relevant literature will demonstrate the extent to which writers have addressed this inclusive vision of palliative care nursing.

Graves and Nash (1992) describe the work of Macmillan nurses, pointing to lack of understanding about their role both by professionals and by lay consumers. In order to explore working patterns, time spent on a number of activities was assessed and check-lists for Macmillan nurses were developed. The significance of these check-lists was seen to lie in their potential for evaluation of nursing provision and they were used by Macmillan nurses in regular reviews of their practice.

Effective timing of visits is important, and must be negotiated in each situation. In morning visits clients were more active and receptive, and a more effective negotiation of objectives took place. Nurses were sensitive to the length of visit, which was determined by the client's condition and how tiring the visit might be. Several other members of the primary healthcare team can also be expected to visit the client, and visits should therefore be necessary and productive, but not too long. The average visit duration was 49 minutes . . . each nurse is left to decide how long to spend on each type of visit, depending on individual knowledge and experience.

Setting out clients' and visit objectives in more detail may make it easier to evaluate the intervention more effectively. It is however, easier to set specific objectives to physical rather than emotional or spiritual needs, but as Stedeford notes: 'No longer overwhelmed by pain and other symptoms, patients become more aware of the emotional and spiritual distress that often accompanies dying'. It is important that such needs are specifically identified.

Graves and Nash (1992) cite the following poignant reflection by a patient, written 6 months before his death, describing his Macmillan nurse:

'This new person in my life
Will take some work on my behalf
(And hers too but she is used to it)
Learning to accept the support
And friendship my brain tells me are vital
But my emotions reject.
It is too soon for me to talk
Of pain relief, home nursing, hospice care.
Please God give me time
To let her establish a relationship

When I can be open and not fight back the tears
To allow her to work with me.'
A poem about a Macmillan nurse written by a client six months before
his death. (Graves and Nash 1992)

The Marie Curie Memorial Foundation is another well-known organization involved in providing palliative nursing services in the UK. The foundation commissioned a comprehensive survey of its community nursing service in 1989 and the report includes a section on the role of the nurse in terminal care. The researchers echoed the view expressed in the article on Macmillan nurses cited above, that 'there is often confusion and misunderstanding about the roles of Marie Curie Community Nurses, District Nurses and Macmillan Nurses' (Owen *et al.* 1989, p. 72). Reviewing a selection of recent publications the authors conclude that the nurse's role has tended to be seen as primarily a traditional bedside caring role, but that there is now a need to extend this concept to incorporate assessment of family needs, co-ordination of care provided by all agencies involved, counselling, and teaching—of both patients and relatives.

A number of authors explicitly addressed nursing behaviours in terminal care. Keith and Castles (1979) conducted a survey of expected and observed behaviour by nurses and patients, based on semi-structured interviews with members of both groups. Instrumental behaviour relates to 'getting the job done', that is, performing specific procedures designed to achieve a certain outcome, for example improved patient comfort. The expressive approach emphasizes emotional support including counselling and provision of advice and support. Patients generally endorsed 'instrumental' behaviour as both the most frequently observed and the most appropriate behaviour for nurses. However, there was also a view that more 'expressive' input would have alleviated the distressing aspects of patients' disease. Waltman and Zimmermann (1991) also studied behavioural intentions by nurses towards dying patients, based on interviews with 372 registered nurses in palliative care. They concluded that, although nurses were likely to provide general nursing care and clear communication with the dying, their continuing support for bereaved relatives was lacking. Degner *et al.* (1991, p. 248) also studied nursing behaviour, based on descriptions by nurse educators and professional nurses of situations when nurses and students had displayed very positive or very negative attitudes to care of the dying. Behaviours identified are summarized in Table 5.1.

Table 5.1   Critical nursing behaviours in care of the dying: operational definitions (Degner *et al.* 1991)

Behaviours	Positive	Negative
Responding during the death scene	Behaviours that maintain a sense of calm	Behaviours that show the nurse's horror of the death scene
Providing comfort	Behaviours that maintain family involvement Behaviours that reduce physical comfort, particularly pain	Controlling behaviour that excludes family Avoidance behaviour that results in neglect Poor symptom management due to poor knowledge base
Responding to anger	Behaviours that show respect and empathy even when anger is directed at nurse	Avoidance behaviour and angry response
Enhancing personal growth	Behaviours that show the nurse has defined a personal role in care for the dying	Behaviours that show anxiety and lack of confidence in care for the dying
Responding to colleagues	Behaviours that provide emotional support and critical feedback to colleagues	Behaviours that show difficulty in providing or receiving support or criticism from colleagues
Enhancing the quality of life during dying	Behaviours that help patients do things that are important to them	Behaviours that show lack of respect for the patient or family
Responding to the family	Behaviours that respond to the family's need for information	Ignoring the family's need for information
	Behaviours that reduce the potential for future regret	Refusing to discuss dying and spiritual issues even when the family clearly wants to do so
	Behaviours that include family in care or relieve them of this responsibility according to what's best for the family	Passing judgment on family decisions and family behaviours toward the dying

The researchers concluded that the lack of clearly defined roles in care of the dying has reinforced a general perception 'that there is nothing left to do'. This study challenges such a view in proposing the development of nursing practice models centred on identified, critical behaviours.

More general approaches to the study of nurses' functions were adopted by a number of writers, addressing these under the headings of: 'characteristics', 'profile', 'work', 'role', and 'model'.

Reisetter and Thomas (1986) discussed the relationship of care for the dying to selected nurse characteristics. 'Avoidance' of the dying patient was identified as an important function of nursing attitudes. The study was based on a mail questionnaire survey of 210 nurses caring for terminally ill patients and a 90% response rate was achieved.

Perhaps no subject in nursing arouses such an emotional response as care of terminally-ill patients. Personal anxieties about death, lack of preparation regarding the care of dying patients and their families, and a professional orientation that emphasizes cure and future health contribute to the nurse's uneasiness with terminally-ill patients. Both theoretical and empirical evidence have established that many nurses, because of their fears and anxieties, often avoid and isolate dying patients. ... Nevertheless, the role of the nurse is central in facilitating peacefulness of death for the patient and resolution of grief for the bereaved. (Reisetter and Thomas 1986)

McCaffrey-Boyle (1994, p. 59) described the 'profiles' of attending nurses, intensivist nurses (intensive care nurses), consulting nurse sub-specialists, and nurse managers. The individual roles of these nurses were outlined. The most relevant aspect of the emerging profiles of all clinical nursing functions listed was the fact that they all included 24 hour responsibility for patients and 'partnership' with physicians, thus stressing a multidisciplinary approach to care.

Deatrick and Fischer (1994) explored the work of oncology nurses, stressing the changing nature of their role. The study was based on phenomenological analysis of accounts given by 38 oncology nurses, describing their daily work. It was concluded that work tended to be variable and there was no concept of a 'typical' day among respondents. Fowler (1994) applied Peplau's model of nursing to palliative care, stressing the dynamic relationship between patient and nurse, which is aimed at promoting 'positive growth'. Gooding *et al.* (1993) demonstrated patient preference for the clinical role of nurses, whereas nurses highlighted empathy as most important. The research was based on comparing the ranking of nurse behaviours by 42 patients and 46 nurses working in Canadian hospital departments of oncology.

It is interesting to note that all but one paper in this sub-section, i.e. that by Fowler, were written by American and Canadian authors, drawing on experiences from their healthcare settings. Fowler described conditions in the UK, but bases the analysis on Peplau's theory which itself comes from the US, thus reinforcing the North American influence on the literature concerning nursing roles in general and, in particular, within the field of palliative care.

Team approaches

The input of palliative care nurses to team work was discussed in a number of papers. Two of these explicitly addressed the nurses' role as team members. McWilliam *et al.* (1993) discussed this issue in the broader context of multidisciplinary collaboration. Although team interaction created some internal and external conflicts among the nurses who formed part of the project, the findings of the study were considered useful in helping all professionals involved to understand the nature of both their own work and that of other team members. Hockley (1992) explored the function of hospital support teams, stressing their role as facilitating rather than 'de-skilling' members of ward teams. Main team functions related to symptom control, emotional and social support of patients and their families, support for staff, education, and research related to palliative care. A question-naire based survey of Canadian palliative care nurses who attended a national conference ($n = 100$) was conducted in the mid 1990s, examining views on various aspects of palliative care, including multidisciplinary teams (Kristjanson and Balneaves 1995). Interest-ingly, respondents expressed concern that development of a separate palliative nursing organization might threaten the interdisciplinary team approach to palliative care. Bromberg and Higginson (1996) conducted a UK-based survey of bereavement follow-up by palliative care teams, exploring views about this service by relatives of patients who had died recently ($n = 320$). The researchers examined bereave-ment follow-up of families by five palliative support teams in the UK. Most carers were spouses (62%). Bereavement follow-up was offered to 215 families (67%). Results of the study indicate the need for improved training of counsellors and clearer protocols setting out chief areas for support in line with identified client needs.

Nursing roles in hospices

As in the previous section, North American literature predominated, with only two papers from the UK. Boyd (1995) studied the working pattern of hospice-based home care teams in the UK, exploring the work patterns of 12 urban hospice teams. The two main alternatives of acting in a mainly participatory or an advisory role were discussed. It was concluded that there is need for review of working patterns of hospice home care team members, considering future models of care provision and defining future objectives for the service. The second article from the UK centred on a comparison between goals in hospice and hospital care (Lunt and Neale 1987). The study was based on interviews with doctors and nurses in two NHS hospices and three medical and two surgical wards in a district general hospital (nurses $n = 50$, doctors $n = 40$). The study revealed the need for better communication between doctors and nurses in the hospital, whereas care goals set by doctors and nurses in the hospices were more complementary. General aspects of hospital care in the US were explored by Daeffler (1985), McGinnis (1986), and Dobratz (1990), who examined general frameworks and overall perspectives supporting hospice nursing. Dobratz views the role of hospice nurses as comprising:

• intensive caring in relation to physical, psychological, social and spiritual problems of dying persons and their families

• collaborative sharing, involving co-ordination and collaboration in all aspects of the extended and expanded hospice services

• continuous knowing, involving acquisition of the counselling, management, instructing, caring, and communication skills needed

• continuous giving, indicating the need for balance between the nurses' self-care needs and the needs of dying people and their families.

Daeffler stressed the nurses' role as assisting dying persons with activities which they are no longer able to perform unaided. Guidelines for hospice nursing should, thus, be structured round

the self-care needs of patients. McGinnis (1986) centred the discussion on nurses' ability to enhance the quality of life of both
hospice residents and their family members, based on an exploratory
study , surveying members of 20 recently bereaved care-giving family
members. The results show preference for nursing behaviours
responding to psychosocial needs related to satisfaction with life,
self-care, and maintenance of control. Sontag (1995) explored
specific characteristics of hospice programs and staff in one
American state. The study sample included 21 chaplains, 95 nurses,
and 27 social workers. Approximately half of the respondents had no
hospice experience prior to their present post. The study provides
background information to guide development of training programmes for hospice staff. Ryan (1992) focused on perspectives
about nursing behaviours in home-based hospice care. Twenty care-
giving, recently bereaved family members and five nurses in a home
care hospice setting completed questionnaires, ranking nurse
behaviours in terms of usefulness. Nurses ranked their role in
teaching carers to deliver physical care and relieve patients'
symptoms as the most important aspect of their role, whereas
care-givers stressed the nurses' role in providing psychosocial
support for patients.

Nursing roles in hospital and the community

The two articles identified as mainly hospital-based both related
to the UK. Krishnasamy (1996) studied nurse behaviour as perceived
by patients treated in an oncology unit specializing in haematology
and bone marrow transplants. Emotionally supportive behaviour by
nurses was generally favoured by patients. (Emotional/psychological
patient and family support will be discussed more fully in a later
section.)

In accordance with findings presented in the literature reviewed, it has
been demonstrated that emotionally supportive behaviour patterns were
identified as being especially helpful by all subjects, with the categories of
reflecting understanding, unconditional availability, respect, intimacy and
companionship being reported as the most supportive nurse behaviour.
(Krishnasamy 1996)

Jupp (1994) described a review of management of care in cancer
wards in a 'major cancer centre'. Findings revealed that a mixture of

team and primary nursing was practised. Primary nursing sometimes failed to utilize every nurse's skills, whereas team nursing facilitated use of capabilities of all staff members.

Two articles specifically addressed community care models. Bergen (1991) reviewed the literature relating to both general district nursing and specialist nursing provision for the terminally ill in the community. The role of the district nurse appeared to be well established and district nurses generally appreciated the specialist service, although there were potential conflicts over responsibility for care. McEnroe (1996), writing about US healthcare, emphasized the identified need for home care oncology nurses to have a broad knowledge base with competency in high technology therapeutic care as well as in more socially oriented care.

Specialist/advanced nursing practice

As noted above there will be no attempt to distinguish between 'specialist' and 'advanced' practice in examining the few articles ($n = 7$) which fell into this category. An uncommonly large and representative sample (baccaleureate nurses $n = 619$ and masters' graduate nurses $n = 637$) was used by McMillan *et al.* (1995) in a study of advanced practice in oncology nursing in the US. Distinction was made between the roles of nurses in what was described as 'basic' compared to 'advanced' practice in oncology nursing. (Conclusions were designed to provide a blueprint for an 'Advanced Oncology Nursing Certification Test' in the US.) Powel and Mayer (1992) explored the future of advanced practice in oncology nursing, which requires masters' degree level education in the US. The authors argued that this function will survive in relation to the ability of advanced practitioners to respond to patient needs. In order to assess their impact there is need to 'define, measure and articulate the effect that advanced practice nurses have on patients with cancer' (p. 28). McCaffrey-Boyle (1995) also examined outcomes of advanced nursing practice based on review of relevant literature, concluding that little research has been undertaken in this area. In order to counteract this paucity theoretical models of advanced nursing practice in oncology need to be developed to support outcome documentation related to such nursing practice. McGee *et al.* (1987) explored specialist competencies of the clinical specialist nurse in oncology, using a Delphi technique. 'Attitudes' and 'human traits' received the highest ratings among the competency categories which were identified by the 47 nurses surveyed. Smith and Waltman (1994) investigated the perceptions of oncology clinical nurse specialists (OCNSs) about their impact on patient outcomes, using a sample of 104 nurses. It was concluded that OCNSs were considered to positively affect both the quality of patient outcomes and costs of the service. A study of 'expert nursing behaviours' in intensive care was conducted by McClement and Degner (1995). They concluded that the most frequently mentioned behaviours by 'nurse experts' in terminal intensive care related prominently to providing emotional support, before and after the death of patients, to patients, relatives, and colleagues. Dicks (1990) stressed the importance of replacing the 'paramedical' model with expert palliative nurses. Holistic care is seen as the ideal approach in which the whole person, rather than just symptoms, is the centre of attention.

The psychological support function and related stress among nurses

The topic of psychological support merits a chapter in its own right and does not fit easily in a discussion about organizational models in palliative care nursing. However, the literature in these areas was too prominent to ignore and it could be argued that the inevitable association between an intensive support function of dying people and the ensuing stress are relevant to the development of appropriate models of nursing in this specialist area. It must, of course, be noted that much stress among nurses relates to other factors which will not be specifically discussed in this paper.

The supportive role of nurses

Davies and Oberle (1990, p. 89) conducted research on the perceptions held by family members of dying patients regarding the nurse's supportive role. Six dimensions were identified:

- valuing
- connecting
- empowering
- doing for

- finding meaning
- preserving own integrity.

Five out of these six dimensions relate to psychological rather than physical aspects of the patient/family–nurse relationship. Hull (1989, 1991) presented a more hard-edged view of the above relationship based on research with families of dying patients. Relevant literature was reviewed in the first paper. The second was based on interviews with and observation of 10 care-giving families in a home based hospice programme. Factual information provided by the nurse was generally preferred to emotional support. Raudonis (1993) explored 'empathy' between nurses and dying patients, based on interviews with 14 terminally ill adults, concluding that understanding the patient's perspective is critical for effective nursing interventions and meaningful outcomes. Cutliffe (1995) reviewed literature on nurses' ability to 'instill hope' in terminally ill patients with HIV and concluded that this related closely to the effectiveness of nursing practice. In a similar vein, Messenger and Roberts (1994) discussed the role of nurses in helping older hospice patients to achieve a state of 'serenity'. The research involved review of relevant literature. Evidence points to the need for nurses to help dying patients to achieve inner peace, which is independent of life events. This is seen to improve patients' quality of life and enhance their spiritual life. Wilson-Barnett (1988) stressed the centrality of 'psychological' and 'comfort' care and the need for the nurse to learn the art of 'coping with the dying'. Hunt (1992) studied conversational interactions between nurses, dying patients and relatives, exploring evidence of shared understanding of the situation. Support for dying patients and relatives in specific situation was discussed by Bakke and Pomietto (1986), Ophof *et al.* (1989), and Mahon (1991). Bakke and Pomietto (1986) addressed the distressing issue of providing support for terminally ill children and their relatives, and responding specifically to psychosocial needs. In their review on care for families of children with late stage cancer, the authors highlight the need to differentiate among various sibling relationships, to emphasize each family member's need for information, to evaluate marital coping behaviours, and to recognize the impact of socioeconomic factors in providing support for grieving families. Ophof *et al.* (1989) discussed the work of a surgical support team in a 'tumour centre' in Heidelberg, Germany, which performed home visits to provide mainly psychological support for patients and relatives. The main conclusion of the research was that home care has clearly improved patients' quality of life. Mahon (1991) explored means of supporting both patients and relatives in coping with the psychosocial consequences of cancer recurrence. Reviewing relevant literature, the author concluded that nurses must first confront their own feelings about the recurrence before being able to assess the needs of patients and relatives realistically. The last article in this section, by Horsley and Brown (1985), provided an appropriate link with the next brief sub-section dealing with stress among nurses. Strengths and needs of US registered and licensed practical nurses and nurses' aides working with hospice patients and relatives were examined. Registered nurses were found to be more confident about aspects of physical care than licensed practical nurses and nurses' aides. They were, however, less confident than the last two groups in the area of providing psychological support.

Stress among palliative care nurses

Only a few key papers from this collection of publications are examined here. Delvaux *et al.* (1988), in reviewing relevant literature, found that working with cancer patients often causes chronic staff stress which can lead to 'burn-out'. The specific stresses of working with dying children were explored by Woolley *et al.* (1989) and Foxall *et al.* (1990) compared perceived job stress experienced by intensive care, hospice, and medical-surgical nurses. A small sample of 18 nurses in a coronary care unit were interviewed about their experience of caring for dying patients. Respondents pointed to the importance of organizational factors as stress relieving, for example an individualized approach to nursing. An egalitarian atmosphere within the nursing team was also viewed as helpful. Continuity of the doctor–nurse relationship on the unit was also rated highly (Field 1989). The real life situation of caring for dying children is described by Woolley (1989b) in the following terms:

The main sources of stress were: the sense of impotence staff felt when they were unable to relieve perceived needs or distress; dealing with negative responses in families, and conflicts within the staff group. The most important mitigating factors were: the informal support that staff provided for each other in this small cohesive working unit, the homelike atmosphere of the hospice, and the diversity of professional and personal skills among the staff group. The implications of these findings for reducing stress among staff dealing with dying people are discussed; this includes not only staff on paediatric wards, intensive care and neonatal units, but also community paediatric nurses.

The area of nurse stress in palliative care and measures taken to relieve it cannot be fully discussed in this chapter, which relates more specifically to the development of models for palliative nursing. However, as management input to stress relief is essential in order for such models to be effective a number of relevant publications on stress and its management will be examined.

Wilson-Barnett (1988b) makes specific reference to the need for 'more supportive managers' of palliative nurses. She also stresses the need for wide-ranging education related to care of the dying and the importance of providing good role models in palliative care nursing. Woolley *et al.* (1989b) also emphasize the need for relevant staff support and training as do Delvaux *et al.* (1988). Management action in this area would appear essential. Owen (1989) addressed the need for 'support groups or meetings or any other form of support' in her survey of Marie Curie nurses. The importance of peer support is also stressed in relation to home-based palliative care by McWilliam *et al.* (1993) and by Davies and Oberle (1990). Such support related to both practical and emotional issues. The need for management support of nurses in stressful situations related to intensive care nursing, hospice nursing and general medical–surgical nursing was emphasized by Foxall *et al.* (1990), noting that stress management programmes must be 'flexible enough to be individualised' (p. 583).

Discussion

This review of literature has as its prime purpose the exploration of valid research data, related to cost-effectiveness and appropriateness of current palliative care services in the NHS. The question focused particularly on nursing concerned with skill-mix and with the cost-effectiveness of specialist roles such as those of specialist and advanced practitioners. These issues are fundamental to effective management of palliative care services and data from the literature will serve as guidance for future policy formation and operational management within this important, but inherently stressful area of care. Managers and research planners also need to take note of important gaps in the available research based literature, for example in relation to cost-effectiveness of nursing services. The fact that most research samples, upon which the literature examined in this paper was based, were small and unrepresentative should also be a matter of concern for managers, in terms of reliability of findings. Identified needs expressed by the main players—patients, family members, and care professionals—should be taken note of by service managers and policy-makers, in order that these can be met in the best possible manner within the prevailing resource constraints.

Skill-mix was not directly addressed in the available literature, but 'role' was substituted as a factor influencing the available combination of nursing skills in the service. Consideration of specialist and advanced practice was made under the same heading.

Although not specifically addressed in the research question, psychological/emotional/spiritual support of dying patients and their relatives formed a major topic in the literature. Stress experienced by nurses related to such support and its management were also commonly reported in published material.

The main areas discussed in the literature will be listed and briefly evaluated, in terms of significance for operational managers and planners of research in palliative care. It should be noted that this discussion does not list all those papers considered in the review. Those selected were deemed to present the most valid data in terms of topic areas, sample size, and representativeness.

- The all-embracing character of palliative care nursing is emphasized by Wilson-Barnett (1988a), stating that 'fundamental' nursing skills are needed in this area.

- Use of specialist palliative nursing services must be cost-effective and well co-ordinated with other nursing services (Owen *et al.* 1989 on Marie Curie nurses and Graves and Nash 1992 on Macmillan nurses).

- Studies of individual nurse behaviour provide valuable insights (Keith and Castles 1979, Degner *et al.* 1991, Waltman and Zimmermann 1991). Individual nurse behaviour and role performance are of crucial importance in team settings as discussed by Hockley (1992), McWilliam *et al.* (1993), Kristjanson and Balneaves (1995), and Bromberg and Higginson (1996).

- Broader perspectives on 'role', 'models' and 'profiles' in palliative nursing are presented by Reisetter and Thomas (1986), Gooding *et al.* (1993), Fowler (1994), McCaffrey-Boyle (1994), and Deatrick and Fischer (1994).

- Nursing roles in specific settings are also described. Hospice nursing was researched by Daeffler (1985), McGinnis (1986), Lunt and Neale (1987), Dobratz (1990), Ryan (1992), Boyd (1995), and Sontag (1995). Palliative nursing specifically in relation to hospital care was discussed by Jupp (1994) and Krishnasamy (1996). Papers by Bergen (1991) and McEnroe (1996) exemplified the debate about the topical area of community-based palliative care. Managers clearly have a fundamental role in assessing the respective benefits of palliative care provided in these different settings, in order to provide the best possible match between the needs of patients and their carers and the available service options.

- Specialist and advanced practitioners constitute an important aspect of palliative care and further studies on the cost-effectiveness of such services are needed. Papers on these topics were published by McGee *et al.* (1987), Dicks (1990), Powel and Mayer (1992), Smith and Waltman (1994), McMillan *et al.* (1995), McCaffrey-Boyle (1995), and McClement and Degner (1995). Management deployment of these expensive services is clearly of great importance.

- The psychological support role of palliative nurses was extensively debated in the literature, both in regard to patients and relatives (Horsley and Brown 1985, Wilson-Barnett 1988, Hull 1989, Ophof *et al.* 1989, Davies and Oberle 1990, Hunt 1991, Raudonis 1993, Messenger and Roberts 1994, and Cutliffe 1995).

- Extensive involvement in providing emotional and psychological support by nurses is likely to produce varying degrees of nurse stress and this must be of concern to managers. A selection of key articles is examined (Delvaux *et al.* 1988, Field 1989, Woolley *et al.* 1989b, and Foxall *et al.* 1990). Management responsibility in stress management is clearly marked in palliative care and relief of nurse stress is discussed by Wilson-Barnett (1988b), Woolley *et al.* (1989b), Delvaux *et al.* (1988), Owen (1989), Davies and Oberle *et al.* (1990), Foxall *et al.* (1990), and McWilliam *et al.* (1993).

Conclusion

In making recommendations for future research in this area of care it is equally important to *build on current strengths* and *identify gaps.,* For example, there is evidence of plentiful and varied research on nurses' role in providing physical and psychological support for patients and relatives, whereas focused research on skill-mix in palliative nursing and on the organization and impact of multi-disciplinary palliative care appear less developed. Financial restraints prompt prior attention to important areas, hitherto comparatively neglected, before areas of strength are further supported. The lack of adequate funding for large scale studies of palliative nursing appears to be a fundamental problem. In the light of these judgments the following recommendations for future research are suggested:

- A concerted attempt should be made by academics, health service managers and policy-makers to achieve more focus on skill-mix and cost-effectiveness in future research and development related to models of palliative care nursing.
- Such research should be based on larger and more representative samples than those available to most researchers whose work has been reviewed in this chapter. This must involve greater access to substantial government or private funding;
- More rigorous techniques should be adopted in palliative nursing research, which combine qualitative and quantitative methods.

Managers have an important role in promoting team work and collaboration between all services involved in palliative care. In this context they are supported by currently available, valid research data, which provide leads for future developments. Collaboration between service managers and academic researchers is essential, enabling them to take joint action in promoting excellence in palliative nursing research and in campaigning for increased funding for this important work. At this time of extending palliative care beyond the traditional association with cancer care it is important that research should cover a wider range of disease groups in terms of palliative care provision for the year 2000 and beyond.

Question 6

Patient and carer satisfaction

EMMA K. WILKINSON

What is known about patient and carer preference for, or satisfaction with, different types of palliative care?

The focus of this review is on consumer preference for, and satisfaction with, different types of palliative care. The term 'consumer' in relation to palliative care generally refers to patients, their families or friends, or informal carers. However, health professionals who seek advice on palliative care matters may also be considered to be 'consumers'(Glickman 1997). Our focus is solely on views of patients and 'informal care-givers' which may include friends, relatives, or spouses but not health professionals. Papers which considered the views of the general public or general attitudes towards palliative care, or the development of research tools to measure satisfaction, were excluded.

Measuring satisfaction

The concept of satisfaction can be operationalized in various ways, and measured using a variety of instruments such as questionnaire or interview surveys. These measures may use direct or open-ended questions and levels of satisfaction may be assessed as global scores or by focusing on specific aspects of care. Researchers may also examine the extent of satisfaction or the intensity/ range of satisfaction. A brief outline of these issues is given below. It is important to note that there is no 'gold standard' for measuring satisfaction (Locker and Dunt 1978).

Patient satisfaction has been regarded as the ultimate validator of the quality of care, and it has been shown to predict patient behaviours related to utilization of health services, continuity with provider, compliance with treatment and advice, and retention and recall of medical information. It is frequently used in formulation of policies to improve the organization of health services. (Fakhoury 1996b)

Impact of wording

Data obtained from surveys can vary substantially, depending on how the questions are framed and when and how the questions are asked (Delbanco 1996). For example, Cohen *et al.* (1996) examined the consistency of the data produced by three interview surveys examining the same aspects of patient dissatisfaction with hospital care. Substantially different results were obtained when asking patients to agree with a negative statement of care as opposed to present-ing them with a positive statement. This highlights the problem of 'response acquiescence' which may be a particular concern in face-to-face interviews when participants may feel under pressure to give socially desirable answers. There is also some evidence that direct questioning about specific issues may elicit different responses. According to Hays and Arnold (1986), direct questioning tends to tap into more general responses to care, whereas the indirect approach assesses more salient beliefs and values.

Response options

The two main approaches to scoring satisfaction include global scores or those which measure differences on specific aspects of care (Locker and Dunt 1978). In general, individual consumers do not hold one overall view of healthcare (Fitzpatrick 1991b). Global measures provide crude measurements which mask the individual consumer's differential preferences for various aspects of health-care. Specific scores use either 'discrete' or 'composite' measures. Composite measures have been criticized for assuming that all items are of equal weighting.

Both global and specific ways of scoring satisfaction may measure either the extent of satisfaction or the range of satisfaction–dissatisfaction (Locker and Dunt 1978). A dichotomous scale is employed for the former and a more sophisticated scale such as a Likert scale for the latter. Measuring the range of satisfaction for specific aspects of care is seen as a more sensitive in detecting variations in intensity of views, but it is notable that interpretation of scores may vary.

Aspects of care

Satisfaction with a variety of aspects of care may be examined and different surveys may examine different components. These may include overall quality, competence, amount of information, bureaucratic arrangements, physical facilities, provider's attention to psychosocial problems of patient, continuity of care, and outcome of care (Higginson 1995a). Researchers have been criticised for focusing on 'hotel aspects of care' such as catering or environment (Glickman 1997). A meta-analysis of 221 studies provided some evidence that aspects of care are measured unevenly (Hall and Dornan 1988).

Assessing satisfaction and consumer opinion

The 'ceiling effect'

One of the main problems in using surveys to assess satisfaction is that results lack variability and the level of satisfaction expressed in surveys tends to be high (Blaxter 1995). It is estimated that at least 80% of respondents will express satisfaction for any given issue (Fitzpatrick 1991b). Criticisms of hospice and specialist palliative care services are particularly rare, owing to their generally high standing in public opinion (Glickman 1997). It is therefore arguable that simple satisfaction surveys alone are likely to be of little practical benefit. This point is clearly illustrated in a survey on hospital care in which satisfaction levels for hospital services were over 89% for most services (Bruster *et al.* 1994). More detailed questioning on patients' experiences revealed a large number of specific problems. To produce meaningful results, consumers views on 'areas for improvement' also need to be elicited (Glickman 1997).

Methodological issues

A key methodological issue is the reliability and validity of data obtained from seriously ill patients or exhausted carers (Moons *et al.* 1994, McWhinney *et al.* 1994). There is some evidence that informal care-givers' reports of patients' experiences may differ from patients' reports of their own experience, particularly in relation to their emotional and physical state (Spiller 1993, Fakhoury *et al.* 1997). The extent to which proxies provide valid accounts of patients' experiences is questionable. Consideration also needs to be paid to the possible ways in which retrospective accounts are subject to change due to the emotional impact of bereavement. There is some evidence that polarization of views of family members may occur after bereavement (Higginson *et al.* 1994a). These issues are discussed in more depth in chapter 5.

Other factors may also influence the validity and reliability of responses. Respondents may feel under pressure to provide socially desirable answers to sensitive questions (Fakhoury *et al.* 1997) especially for medical care which they have personally received (Fakhoury *et al.* 1996c). The reluctance of recipients of care to express negative answers is well documented. Also responses may be altered as a function of being observed and may not reflect the respondents' 'real' opinions ('Hawthorne effect'). Similarly, positive first impressions of one aspect of care may distort consumers' views of other aspects of care ('halo effect'). Interviewer variability may also influence responses and interviewers' own interpretations of respondents' views.

Theoretical limitations

The concept of 'satisfaction' is rarely defined *a priori* in research, as authors assume that most people know its meaning (Wilkinson 1986). The meaning to researchers and respondents generally has received little attention (Locker and Dunt 1978) and no well-defined consensus theory of satisfaction exists (Hays and Arnold 1986, Wilkinson 1986). It is therefore arguable that satisfaction may be defined differently by patients, staff, and families depending on their previous experience and their own evaluations of aspects of care.

Another theoretical criticism of consumer surveys is that they reflect the conceptual bias of the provider rather than the consumer (Blaxter 1995). The view that patients or their families have a limited outlook in terms of their knowledge of medical care or of the full range of alternatives has also been a source of criticism for satisfaction surveys (Blaxter 1995).

Determinants of satisfaction

Few consistent associations have been found between satisfaction and demographic variables, with the exception of age. Generally, respondents over the age of 65 are less likely to express dissatisfaction (Blaxter 1995, Fakhoury *et al.* 1996c). Recent work by Fakhoury *et al.* (1996b, 1996c, 1997) has identified several non-service and service determinants of informal care-giver satisfaction. In a retrospective study of 1858 informal care-givers' of deceased cancer patients, it was found that the frequency of visits by district nurses and general practitioners as well as the provision of information regarding diagnosis were all powerful predictors of informal care-giver satisfaction with care services (Fakhoury *et al.* 1996b). In terms of non-service predictors of satisfaction, there was some evidence for an association between site of cancer and satisfaction with hospital care (Fakhoury 1997). In another study, some patient and informal care-giver attributes were found to be highly predictive of informal care-giver satisfaction with services (Fakhoury *et al.* 1996c). Informal care-givers who perceived caring as rewarding, who had no unmet needs while caring for patients at home, and those who expressed a positive health status post-bereavement, were more likely than others to be satisfied. Carers whose patients were functionally incapacitated shortly before death were less satisfied. Overall, these results highlight the importance of consideration of patient and informal care-giver characteristics in the interpretation of results from satisfaction surveys.

In spite of the potential limitations of research into patient and carer satisfaction with healthcare, the value of this research should not be overlooked. It can be valuable in terms of understanding and predicting consumer behaviour including advice seeking, compliance with regimes, assessing patterns of communication between consumers and providers, and helping to decide between alternative ways of organizing healthcare (Fitzpatrick 1991b). The unique vantage point of patients and their families can serve to make important suggestions as well as describe what is and is not going well.

Evidence from the literature review

The vast majority of the studies on consumer preference and satisfaction with various models of palliative were based in the UK or North America. Given the difficulties in making meaningful comparisons between palliative care services which differ historically, structurally, and functionally, findings from studies based in the UK are considered separately from those based in North America. Only a small number of studies from mainland Europe focused on consumer views on palliative care. (Eriscsson Persson *et al.* 1984, Petrosino 1985, Dawson 1991, Petersen 1992, Merrouche *et al.* 1996). As the focus of these studies varied and they were 'scattered' across five countries, their results are not discussed. Only a handful of studies examined paediatric palliative care and as these varied in quality, focus, and setting they were also excluded from the discussion below (Edwardson 1983, Lauer *et al.* 1983, Delight and Goodall 1988, Stein *et al.* 1989,Woolley *et al.* 1989a, Duffy *et al.* 1990).

In-patient hospice care in the UK: satisfaction and opinions

Comparative studies on opinions of in-patient hospice versus in-patient hospital care

Comparative studies in the late 1970s which have specifically compared hospice care to hospital care have generally indicated that hospice care was viewed more favourably than hospital care especially with regard to psychosocial aspects of care (Parkes 1979, Hinton 1979). Consumer reports that hospice care provide better pain control than general hospitals have proved inconsistent, although there is no evidence that this aspect of care was viewed as inadequate or worse than hospital care. Indeed, there is some evidence from consumer reports that pain control has generally improved in both hospice and hospital settings (Parkes and Parkes 1984). This is a key issue, as pain control has found to be a prime concern of patients on admission to institutional care (McDonnell 1989).

   Hinton (1979) examined differences in consumer opinion in four different care environments including in-patient and out-patient hospice care, general hospital care,and a foundation home. Hospice patients reported lower levels of depression and anxiety compared to foundation home patients. Opinions on physical care, communication, and place of care were generally positive across all environments. Hospice care was viewed more favourably than other settings in terms of patients feeling less troubled. Patients gave most praise to out-patient systems of hospice care, above all other types of care including in-patient hospice care. However, a potential limitation of this study is that the results are based on interviewers' own ratings of patients and carers' views. Another study also found opinions favouring in-patient hospice care at St Christopher's Hospice over local hospital care (Parkes 1979). In comparison to Hinton's study, the hospice in-patients reported lower levels of pain than those in the hospital in-patient group. Patients reported experiencing lower levels of distress and spouses of hospice patients also reported less anxiety and being able to spend more time with the patient than did their hospital counterparts.

No great benefit of pain control was found in a follow-up study comparing hospice care at St Christopher's hospice to local hospital care (Parkes and Parkes 1984). However, other aspects of hospice care were viewed more favourably. Indeed, surviving spouses of both hospital cancer patients and hospice cancer patients were significantly less concerned about patient pain and distress and also showed less bereavement stress during the period 1977–79 in comparison with views expressed by cohorts of surviving spouses in 1967–69.

Comparative studies on satisfaction with in-patient hospice care versus conventional care

Two studies published in the early 1990s indicated that satisfaction with in-patient hospice care is generally high. These studies provide some evidence that consumers are more satisfied with hospice care than conventional care, although some methodological flaws and the general 'patchiness' of evidence undermine the certainty of this conclusion. Indeed, a retrospective study by Seale (1991b) examined views on care across 14 in-patient hospices in comparison with conventional care. Surviving relatives' of hospice patients reported significantly more favourable views on nursing care and care in general than the conventional care group, although no differences were found between the two groups in terms of satisfaction with site of death. It is notable that the hospice patients had fewer medical problems but worse symptoms than the conventional care group of patients. The potential effect of these medical differences on results is difficult to determine. A relatively small-scale study by Field *et al.* (1992) examined satisfaction levels of 59 informal care-givers of patients who had experienced conventional care prior to receiving hospice care at the Leicestershire hospice. Informal care-givers were satisfied with care received in hospice, but somewhat less satisfied with care received by community doctors and nurses in comparison with hospice staff.

Summary

Overall, comparative studies examining consumer views on in-patient hospice care with hospital care or conventional care are limited. Indeed, not only have relatively few studies examined these types of care, most have concentrated on hospice care provided by St Christopher's hospice (Parkes 1979, Parkes and Parkes 1984). The fact that many findings were based on care from one site may limit the generalizability of these results. However, the lack of spont-aneous criticism reported across all studies involving hospice care is notable. Indeed, only Field's study indicated that a few minor complaints were made. Positive comments were more forthcoming and mainly indicated patients' and carers' appreciation of the non-clinical aspects of care. Favourable aspects of in-patient hospice care included the humaneness of care (Seale 1991b), the reduction of anxiety (Hinton 1979, Parkes 1979, Parkes and Parkes 1984), open and honest communication (Parkes 1979), and supportive nursing care (Seale 1991b).

Hospice home care services in the UK: satisfaction and opinions

Consumer opinion of hospice home care services

Only a small number of studies have examined consumer views on hospice home care services. It is therefore difficult to draw firm conclusions, especially as the findings are likely to lack external validity. Non-comparative studies have highlighted the perceived benefits of home care, including 24-hour access to professional care (Hinton 1996) and attention to symptom control (Hinton 1994a). However, the need for more complementary in-patient care has been highlighted (Hinton 1994a).

The types of care that patients and relatives mainly saw as helpful were medication, physical nursing help and a spectrum of supportive psycho-logical activities, including staff just keeping in touch. (Hinton 1996)

Further advantages and disadvantages of hospice home care were highlighted by Parkes (1980). He examined the views of surviving spouses of cancer patients who had received home care provided by St Christopher's Hospice (which provided advice and assessment only), compared to the views of surviving spouses of cancer patients who had experienced ordinary home care. Reports made by spouses 13 months after the death of patients indicated that patients who had received special home care had been able to stay at home until a later stage in their illness and also spent less time in hospital. However, home care patients felt more of a burden and showed greater feelings of tension, and spouses of these patients also reported experiencing greater anxiety while the patient was at home. The extent to which these findings truly reflect the impact of home hospice care is limited by the fact that patients in the St Christopher's group had greater nursing needs than those in the control group.

Specialist outreach teams in the community: satisfaction and opinions

Comparative studies examining satisfaction with specialist home care services for people with HIV/AIDS indicate that they compare favourably with other community care services (McCann 1991) and also with primary and secondary services (Higginson *et al.* 1990, Butters *et al.* 1993). Indeed, McCann (1991) found that people with HIV/AIDS rated the community team as significantly more kind and understanding than general practitioners, and their overall care was rated more highly. Patients believed that the support team's key functions were to provide reassurance, support, and advice. Butters *et al.* (1993) found that although people with HIV/AIDS and their lay carers were more satisfied with the community care team than with the services provided by primary or secondary care, they were un-clear of the role of the community care team. The fact that the patients who were interviewed had lower levels of pain, less anxiety, and better insight than those who were not interviewed may underlie these positive results. Similarly, in a comparison of cancer patients' views on community-based support teams, general community and hospital care, most praise was given to the community-based support teams and least to hospital doctors and nurses (Higginson *et al.* 1990).

Consumer opinions on 'home' as a site of death

Findings from several studies support the notion that 'home' as the site of death is generally preferred (Brown *et al.* 1990, Addington

Hall *et al.* 1991, Sykes *et al.* 1992, Hinton 1994a). An interview study of 80 family carers whose relatives had experienced either home care or acute general hospital care found that home carers were significantly more satisfied with the site of death than the carers of those who died in hospital (Addington Hall *et al.* 1991). Brown *et al.* (1990) found that cancer patients and their families preferred home care to hospital or nursing home care as they were able to continue with established patterns of interaction which enabled some control over daily routines and also enabled them to maintain a level of normality in their lives. The nature of some hospice home care services may also contribute to this preference, as patients can have 24-hour access to specialized support (Hinton 1996). The increasing availability of specialized care at home may have contributed to consumer preference for dying at home. However, it is notable that preference for home care may fluctuate according to the stage of terminal illness of the patient (Hinton 1994a).

In spite of consumer preference for home care as a site of death, several studies indicate that in practice consumer preference was not realised as patients did not actually die in a setting of their choice. An interview survey of 84 cancer patients found that 58% wished to die at home, but only 29% did so. Although only 20% of patients wished to die in hospital, 54% did so (Townsend *et al.* 1990). Sykes *et al.* (1992) noted that of 100 deaths which occurred in hospital and at home, 91% of informal care-givers whose relatives died at home were present at death compared to only 40% of carers whose relatives died in hospital. Barriers to choosing the 'home' as the site of death generally relate to a perceived lack of resources, particularly with regard to nursing and medical care (Brown *et al.* 1990, Townsend *et al.* 1990).

In-patient hospital care and non-specialist care in the community: satisfaction and opinions

Comparative studies on consumer views on hospital versus community care

This section specifically examines views on and satisfaction with in-patient hospital care compared to general community services. The earliest comparative study of hospital care with ordinary home care, in the late 1970s, found that although hospital patients dying from cancer experienced less pain than their home care counterparts, they were also less active and conscious than their home care counterparts (Parkes 1978). Although these findings have not been replicated since, studies in the 1980s and 1990s have indicated that consumers have reported a wide range of problems with in-patient hospital care.

Wilkes (1984) examined 262 carers' retrospective views on hospital and home care received by their relatives. Although care received by almost a third of patients who had received hospital care was praised, almost a quarter of relatives criticized the uncaring attitude of hospital care and complained of poor symptom control and of difficulties in extracting information from doctors. Criticisms of the home care group focused on infrequent general practitioner visits and difficulties in access to care and equipment, although the skills and support provided by general practitioners were praised.

In a comparison of cancer patients' views on community-based support teams, general community care, and hospital care, least praise was given to hospital doctors and nurses and most to the community-based support teams (Higginson *et al.* 1990). Communication was seen as a key problem in both primary and secondary care and further complaints were made about the co-ordination of services and perceptions of hospital doctors being overworked.

Comparative studies on satisfaction with hospital care versus general community care

An interview study of 80 family carers whose relatives had experienced either home care, acute general hospital or in-patient hospice care found consumers were more dissatisfied with hospital care compared to care in the other settings (Addington-Hall *et al.* 1991). Approximately half of the carers whose patients had experienced hospital care were dissatisfied with care and 39% were dissatisfied with information received from the hospital. In comparison, just under a third were dissatisfied with the care received from general practitioners. Similarly, Fakhoury *et al.* (1996b) found that informal care-givers were more dissatisfied with hospital care compared with community care. Informal care-givers were more highly satisfied with district nursing services compared to those delivered by either hospital doctors or general practitioners.

[with regard to] hospital services, two-fifths of carers were dissatisfied with the amount of information patients and families were given—and with the way it was given. In particular, some carers felt that they had not been given enough information about the timing of death. ... The unsuitability of acute wards for dying patients emerged ... as a cause of dissatisfaction with hospital care. Nurses were often reported to be doing their best but, due to lack of time, were unable to give dying patients the care and attention they needed. (Addington-Hall *et al.* 1991)

A more recent study by McCarthy *et al.* (1997a) indicated varying satisfaction levels with primary and secondary palliative care, as experienced by consumers suffering from different terminal illnesses. An interview survey of the views of the informal carers of both dementia and cancer patients with regard to hospital and general practitioner care found that dementia patients were slightly more dissatisfied with hospital care and general practitioner care than cancer patients. In particular, 34% of respondents for dementia patients found the hospital room for their patient as 'not at all peaceful and quiet' compared to only 22% of cancer patient carers. Over a third of dementia patient respondents and over a half of cancer patient respondents complained of being unable to obtain enough information in hospitals. Although general practitioner care was rated as excellent or good by most respondents, fewer dementia patients' respondents (50%) thought the general practitioner was very understanding compared to 60% of cancer patients.

Non-comparative studies on hospital care for non-cancer patients

Several non-comparative studies have examined satisfaction with hospital care for non-cancer patients. A retrospective study by Addington-Hall *et al.* (1995) found that many informal carers were dissatisfied with hospital care for stroke patients. A sizeable minority criticized hospital facilities, as 27% thought that patients were not given enough privacy, and 18% believed the room was not at all peaceful or quiet. Approximately one third of carers believed that care was too rushed and that patients had little choice, and 39% of informal care-givers were unable to obtain information about the patient's condition. Another retrospective study examining consumer opinions on hospital care for patients with cardiovascular disease (McCarthy *et al.* 1996). Over 80% of informal care-givers rated the care of hospital doctors and nurses as good or excellent, in spite of poor symptom control.

Non-comparative studies on general community care

Only a handful of small-scale, non-comparative studies in this review focused on satisfaction with non-specialist palliative care in the community (Sykes *et al.* 1992, Cowley 1993, Jones *et al.* 1993). These studies were variable in quality and their focus was on different aspects of community care. Rather than compare satisfaction levels across these studies, a more fruitful approach would be to examine areas in which consumers believed community care was working well and where improvements may be required. Jones *et al.* (1993) found that although 94% of informal care-givers of deceased cancer patients rated home care support as excellent or good, 60% reported not receiving advice on financial support, and 84% reported that they were not informed of local support from charities. Others have also found a lack of awareness of the nature and availability of services in the community (Cowley 1993). Sykes *et al.* (1992) found that 10% of 47 family care-givers were dissatisfied with community services and that reasons for dissatisfaction related to the unhelpful attitudes of health professionals, lack of unsolicited support, and lack of practical help with physical problems.

Summary

Consumer views on the palliative care received from general hospitals are generally more critical than those relating to all types of hospice care or to specialist care in the community. Criticisms of hospital care are not only numerous, but are also wide-ranging. Difficulties in obtaining appropriate information in hospitals were cited in several studies (Wilkes 1984, Hockley *et al.* 1988, Addington-Hall *et al.* 1991, McCarthy *et al.* 1997a). Another frequently mentioned problem involved consumer perceptions that hospital staff were too busy (Higginson *et al.* 1990, Addington-Hall *et al.* 1991, Hull 1991) or lacked time to discuss medical issues (Addington-Hall *et al.* 1995, Hockley *et al.* 1988). Other concerns about the hospital environment focused on the lack of privacy or peace and quiet (McCarthy *et al.* 1997a). Further criticisms related to a lack of adequate co-ordination between primary and secondary care services

(Higginson *et al.* 1990). However, it is notable that two relatively recent randomized controlled trials have found no effect of co-ordinating care for terminally ill cancer patients on satisfaction levels (Addington Hall *et al.* 1992, MacDonald *et al.* 1994).

Although these studies indicate a large number of concerns with regard to palliative care in secondary care centres, they do not reflect the majority view, rather that of a sizeable minority. Furthermore, the extent to which these concerns apply to both cancer and non-cancer patients is difficult to determine. Given that there is some evidence that the treatment of cancer and non-cancer patients differs, at least with regard to the provision of information on diagnosis and prognosis (Zylicz 1996), more research is required to understand the specific ways in which their experiences may differ or overlap.

Consumer views about community care have also highlighted several specific areas for concern. These difficulties included a lack of access to specialist services or equipment (Wilkes 1984, Higginson *et al.* 1990, Jones *et al.* 1993) and problems with out of hours care (Addington Hall *et al.* 1991). Other concerns included difficulties with physical care (Sykes *et al.* 1992, Jones *et al.* 1993) and a lack of awareness of the full range of available options for care (Cowley 1993, Jones *et al.* 1993).

In-patient hospice care in North America: satisfaction and opinions

Comparative studies on satisfaction with in-patient hospice care versus conventional care

In North America, studies of patient and carer satisfaction with in-patient hospice care compared to more conventional forms of care have reaped inconsistent results. Drawing any firm conclusions has also proved difficult, owing to some methodological flaws in studies and the focus on satisfaction with different aspects of care. The National Hospice Study (Greer *et al.* 1986), examined carer and patient satisfaction across 40 hospices and 14 conventional care centres. Satisfaction with hospital-based hospice care, hospice home care, and conventional care were compared. No differences were found in levels of satisfaction between groups, and satisfaction levels were above 90% in all settings. Family members of patients receiving both types of hospice care reported greater satisfaction with care

Table 6.1 Comparative studies on patient or lay carer opinions or satisfaction with various types of palliative care in the UK

Authors	Study design(s)	Intervention	Subjects[a]	Outcome measures	Results	Conclusions	Comments
McCarthy et al. (1997a)	Interview survey	Investigation of the experience of dying for people with terminal cancer and end-stage dementia during last year of life. (From lay carer perspective)	Random sample of dementia and cancer patients over the age of 65 at death. (Randomly chosen from 20 health districts). Total no. 1683 2 conditions: dementia (n = 170) cancer (n = 1513)	Carer satisfaction Morbidity Patient/carer/ professional's opinion Provision of care needs	75% of dementia group and 72% of cancer group thought general practitioner care was excellent or good 50% of dementia group compared to 60% for cancer rated the general practitioner as very understanding No significant differences between 2 groups on satisfaction with residential care 34% of dementia group described hospital room that the patient had spent most time in as 'not at all peaceful and quiet' compared to 22% of cancer group 39% of dementia group were unable to get all information required on patient's condition, compared to 51% of respondents for cancer 35% of dementia patients' informal carers found care rewarding compared to 60% of cancer cases Dementia patients were less frequently hospitalized, but spent more time in hospital	Respondents for dementia patients slightly more satisfied with care than were cancer patients. Lay carers also found care less rewarding	Random sample of patients Study uses carers as a proxy for patients Retrospective

Table 6.1 (contd)

Authors	Study design(s)	Intervention	Subjects[a]	Outcome measures	Results	Conclusions	Comments
Seamark (1996)	Retrospective interview or questionnaire survey	Comparison of quality of care in community hospitals with care in hospice	Lay carers ($n = 161$) of patients who had died of cancer (NB 106 interviewed, 55 questionnaires) Hospice ($n = 70$) Hospitals ($n = 91$)	Carer opinion	Lay carers found professionals in hospices easier to talk to compared to those in community hospitals ($p < 0.05$) Lay carers in the hospice group significantly more likely to be present at the time of death than those of community hospital patients ($p < 0.0001$) Lay carers in the community hospital group reported more negative comments than those in the hospice group. Criticisms focused on problems of communication, lack of nursing staff and lack of support in bereavement	Over 90% of lay carers assessed terminal care as good or excellent, despite criticisms regarding communication, lack of nursing staff and bereavement support. Hospice care attracted less criticism	From lay carers' perspective, interviewed 4–6 weeks after patients' death
Butters et al. (1993)	Interview survey Questionnaire survey	Views on palliative care provided by home care team. After 3–4 weeks of care and also at 4–6 weeks. Patients vs. informal	People with HIV/AIDS, majority were homosexual, all had live-in carers Of 125 patients, only 19 were interviewed (all were rated on STAS by CCT)	Carer satisfaction Morbidity Patient satisfaction	After 3–4 weeks of care by Community Care Team (CCT) symptom control was identified as most severe problem. Other problems: pain control, family and patient anxiety, problems with communication with other professionals. 18/19 patients and carers rated CCT's care as good or excellent,	Patients and carers generally satisfied with CCT and less content with care of primary and secondary services	Conclusions may be limited by sample bias. Unable to interview 105/125 AIDS patients due to ill health. Patients

Study	Focus	Methods	Measures	Findings	
	care-givers vs. community care team views	Interviews with 19 lay carers and 19 patients; 19 ratings by CCT (Ratings compared on the Support Team Assessment Schedule)		although they were not completely clear of the role of the CCT Patients and carers' negative comments focused on communication problems with general practitioners, hospital doctors, and nurses in discussing diagnosis, prognosis, their attitude and difficulties getting through to CCT out of hours	interviewed experienced fewer problems and may be more satisfied with care as a result
Field *et al.* (1992)	Comparison of community care with hospice care Comparison of lay carer views of care before and 3 months after death	hospice patients (details of disease not given) Total no: 59 Lay carers interviewed on admission Lay carers re-interviewed after patient death(*n* = 37)	Carer satisfaction Patient satisfaction Carers' opinion	Lay carers rated 63% of nurses as giving 'a lot' or 'some' reassurance and support compared to 46% of general practitioners. Lay carers were significantly more likely to rank hospice nurses care as 'excellent' than community nurses ($p < 0.001$) 38% of general practitioners care was rated 'good' or 'excellent' compared to 63% for community nurses. No significant differences in ratings of care of hospice doctors and general practitioners Lay carers significantly less likely to rate care they themselves received from hospice staff as highly as they rated care given to patients ($p < 0.001$) Lay carers rated 89% of hospice staff as 'willing to give information' although 54% of carers felt they had to ask for information	Lay carers were more satisfied with hospice care than community care Patient's levels of satisfaction with hospice staff were higher than lay carers Over half of lay carers had to actively seek information from hospice staff and relatively few (*n* = 9) received bereavement follow-up care

Table 6.1 (contd)

Authors	Study design(s)	Intervention	Subjects[a]	Outcome measures	Results	Conclusions	Comments
Seale (1991a)	Retrospecive interview survey	Comparison of hospice care (including in-patient care and home care) with conventional care during last year of life	Random sample of cancer patients age 15 or over. Total no.: 171 Hospice ($n = 45$) Conventional care ($n = 126$)	Carer opinion Morbidity	Hospice patients had fewer conditions (other than cancer), worse symptoms and more restrictions of daily activities 92% of hospice group responded that hospice nurses had given a lot of reassurance and support, compared to only 69% of conventional care group (re: care given by district nurses) 96% of respondents considered nursing care during in-patient stay as excellent, compared to only 57% of conventional care respondents 91% of hospice respondents considered doctors' care 'excellent', compared to 40% of conventional care respondents No difference between 2 groups on satisfaction levels with site of death 100% of hospice respondents described hospice staff support at time of death as 'very kind and understanding' compared to 83% of conventional care respondents	Satisfaction with hospice care was generally higher compared to conventional care Key aspects of hospice care most valued included: reassurance and support provided by hospice nurses, and the caring, supportive atmosphere of hospices and attention to symptom control	Weaknesses: significant medical differences between the two groups, and use of relatives views as proxy Strengths: 14 hospices involved in study

McCann (1991)	Interview survey	Comparison of patients views' on Home Support Team (HST) with general practitioner care and out-patient care	People with AIDS, mainly homosexual, all male. 42% had known about HST for over 1 year and 25% less than 6 months. Majority still worked full time. Total no: 261 2 main groups: HST ($n=119$) Control ($n=142$)	Patient satisfaction Utilization of healthcare	78% of HST patients thought staff were kind and understanding; these ratings slightly higher than for social workers (73%) and out-patient staff (74%) and significantly higher than general practitioner care (49%) ($p<0.001$). (NB different numbers of patients used each service) 49% rated HST care as excellent and 37% as 'v. good' and this was significantly different to ratings for general practitioners ($p<0.05$.) Majority of patients believed the HST provided either a lot of reassurance and support, (60%), or some reassurance and support (31%). Much of the support teams work was seen as giving advice, and the majority found it very helpful, (64%), or fairly helpful,(26%)	People with AIDS viewed the HST care in a positive way, especially in terms of offering support; their views on this type of care compared favourably to other forms of care including social work, out-patient and general practitioner care in particular Strengths: 1) Prospective study. 2) Patients' own views
Addington-Hall et al. (1991)	Interview survey	Comparison of care received during last week of life. Home care versus hospice versus hospital	Terminally ill cancer patients, expected to live for 1 year or less Total no: 80 family carers of patients 3 main conditions: Home care ($n=31$) Hospital care ($n=41$)	Carer satisfaction Morbidity Carer opinion	97% of carers of patients who died at home were satisfied with place of death, compared with 53% of those who died in hospital ($p<0.01$) Half of carers of patients who received hospital care were dissatisfied (37/73) mainly due to fact that nurses were too busy to provide adequate care. 27% of 64 carers who had	Although family carers appreciated nursing and medical care for terminally ill cancer relatives, areas of dissatisfaction were identified and included:

Table 6.1 (contd)

Authors	Study design(s)	Intervention	Subjects[a]	Outcome measures	Results	Conclusions	Comments
			Hospice care (n = 8)		contact with general practitioners during final illness were dissatisfied although 2/3 were satisfied and 2/3 thought care was well co-ordinated. 39% of carers were dissatisfied with information received from hospital. 20% of carers who had contact with district nurses were dissatisfied due to lack of continuity of care. In last week of life, over 50% of patients suffered from pain, dyspnoea, insomnia and depression and 20% received no effective treatment for pain.	inadequate symptom control, undesirable nature of dying on busy acute wards, difficulties in obtaining information and lack of community services and out of hours support	
Higginson et al. (1990)	Prospective interview survey	Evaluation of community based support teams' services and hospital and community services from family and patient perspective	Terminally ill cancer patients, mean age 66 years, all with a family carer. Total no: 65 participants	Patient and carer opinion	Support teams received most praise by patients (89%) and family (91%) 71% of family and 71% of patients rated general practitioner care and district nurses' care as good or excellent, compared to 34% of patients and 54% of family who rated care of hospital doctors and nurses at this level Negative comments on care of hospital staff focused on communication, co-ordination of	Support teams were praised by the majority of families and patients. Primary care rated more favourably than secondary care Poor communication was identified as	Weaknesses: No control Strengths: Prospective i.e. views of carers and patients before death

Parkes and Parkes (1984)	Retrospective interview survey	Comparison of hospice care with hospital care. Also comparison of care in 1967–69 with care in 1977–79 (Care from perspective of surviving spouse)	Patients who had died of cancer In 1967–69: hospice ($n = 34$) hospital ($n = 34$) In 1977–79: hospice ($n = 30$) hospital ($n = 30$) (matched pairs)			
					services, and being too overworked to care Complaints for primary care were on communication (at diagnosis esp.), attitude, and difficulties in getting general practitioners to do home visits Patients and families rated symptom control as most severe problem, although families rated this problem (and pain control and effect of anxiety) as significantly worse than patients ($p < 0.05$.)	most common problem in primary and secondary care
				Carers opinion Morbidity	Over 10 years (from 1969–79) anxiety decreased in both groups. In the 1977–79 groups, levels of anxiety were significantly less for those cared for at St Christopher's Hospice, compared to those cared for in local hospitals ($p < 0.05$) Spouses believed patients suffered less overall pain ($p < 0.05$) and severe distress ($p < 0.05$) in 1977–79, compared to 1967–69 (in both hospital and hospice groups) Post-bereavement stress and grief experienced by surviving spouses significantly less in 1977–79 compared to 1967–69 ($p < 0.05$ St Christopher's, $p < 0.002$ local hospitals) in both groups	Spouses of patients were less concerned about pain and distress suffered by patients in 1977–9 compared to 1967–9 and less anxious during this period under care of St Christopher's hospice compared to local hospital care. Findings attributed to greater involvement of spouses in hospice care

Weaknesses: Statistical results not presented clearly; closed questionnaire Strength: Matched pairs

Table 6.1   (contd)

Authors	Study design(s)	Intervention	Subjects[a]	Outcome measures	Results	Conclusions	Comments
Wilkes (1984)	Retrospective interview survey	Comparison of carers' views on hospital versus home care	Patients who died of heart disease (38%), cancer (32%), and stroke (12%) Total no: 262 deceased patients	Views of nurses, general practitioners, community nurses and relatives	Relatives reported difficulties with home care especially in obtaining medical help at night from a doctor who knew patient and in obtaining equipment on time 24% of relatives praised general practitioners skills and support, although 37% complained of infrequency of home visits. 27% of relatives criticized uncaring nature of hospital care; other criticisms focused on differences in extracting information, poor symptom control and overtreatment Relatives praised hospital care in 29% of cases, 34% praising hospital nurses more than any other professionals Relatives and health professionals held different perceptions of problems of patients	Relatives praised care provided by hospital nurses more than any other professional. Difficulties in unreliable home care services and the uncaring nature of hospital services were put forward by a sizeable minority of relatives	
Parkes (1980)	Retrospective interview survey	Comparison of St Christopher's Home Care Team versus	Married men or women who died of cancer under the age of 70. Surviving spouses	Carers opinion	Patients in St Christopher's group more seriously ill and felt more of a burden ($p < 0.02$) Surviving relatives in hospice group reported experiencing greater	Surviving relatives were positive about help received from St	Strengths: Matched pairs in terms of age, sex, severity of

	Design	Aim	Sample	Measures	Results	Conclusions	Strengths/Weaknesses
		ordinary home care	Interviewed 13 months after death Total no: 102 surviving spouses St Christopher's home care ($n = 51$) Ordinary home care ($n = 51$) (matched pairs)		anxiety while patient was in their care ($p < 0.01$) Patients in St Christopher's group stayed at home until a later stage in illness Surviving relatives expressed positive feelings about help received from home care service. 100% reported improvements in patient's peace of mind and 97% in their own Spouses of patients ($n = 23$) from St Christopher's group who were admitted into hospital to die reported significantly more positive feelings than spouses of patients ($n = 23$) in control group in same situation	Christopher's Home Care Service, although it did not reduce their stress levels or need for primary care help. Patients in the St Christopher's group had greater nursing needs than control group.	pain before terminal period etc. Weaknesses: Significant medical differences between groups
Hinton (1979)	Prospective interview survey	Comparison of care provided in four environments: general hospital, foundation home, hospice (in-patient) and hospice (out-patient); during last three months of life.	Cancer patients, both male and female, all married Total no: 80 general hospital ($n = 20$) foundation home ($n = 20$) hospice in-patient ($n = 20$) hospice out-patient ($n = 20$)	Patient/carer/ professional's opinion Psychological status	Patients' opinions on physical care, staff, communication with nurses, and place of care were all positive Observer ratings show hospice in-patients were 'less troubled', and less depressed compared to patients in acute hospital and in the cancer care home. No consistent significant differences in ratings between Foundation Home and acute hospital wards were found. Patients favoured more open communication. Hospice out-patients significantly	Patients gave most praise to out-patient systems of care in spite of experiencing slightly more anxiety. Patients were least distressed in a hospice environment and showed preference for open communication	Strengths: Prospective study Weaknesses: Ratings made by interviewer, while conducting interview. No pre-set criteria for observation.

Table 6.1 (contd)

Authors	Study design(s)	Intervention	Subjects[a]	Outcome measures	Results	Conclusions	Comments
Parkes (1979)	Retrospective interview survey	Comparison of hospital care with in-patient hospice care, from perspective of surviving spouse (interviewed 13 months after bereavement)	Patients who died from cancer under age of 65 Total no: 68 surviving spouses of patients Hospital ($n = 34$) Hospice group ($n = 34$)	Carer opinion	more anxious, angry and depressed compared to hospice in-patients. Patients at hospice reported to suffer less severe pain and distress than patients in hospital group $p < 0.05$. Hospice group remained more mobile than hospital group, with 39% not confined to bed compared to 13%. $p < 0.05$. 36% of hospice patients fully aware of prognosis compared to 18% of hospital patients. Surviving spouses in hospice group likely to spend more time with patient ($p < 0.001$) and talk more to members of staff, compared to spouses in other group ($p < 0.01$). Nurses, ward sisters and doctors at hospice seen as less busy than those at hospitals. Surviving spouses in hospice reported less anxiety ($p < 0.01$), and were less worried about patient's suffering physical pain ($p < 0.01$)	In-patient hospice care was reported to be more effective than hospital care by surviving spouses of patients in terms of providing more effective pain control and patients being more mobile and more fully aware of prognosis than hospital patients	Strengths: Matched pairs and no significant differences between groups

[a] Total number and number per condition.

before and after death and with place of death than did their counterparts receiving conventional care. The generalizability of these results may be limited by the unrepresentative nature of the sites of care. Also, some inconsistency in the application of selection criteria for patient undermines the reliability of these results.

In contrast to the findings of the National Hospice Study, a randomized controlled trial found that hospice patients were significantly more satisfied with hospice care than were conventional care patients with their care (Kane *et al*. 1984). In particular, patients were more satisfied with qualitative aspects of care, i.e. involvement and interpersonal care. No differences were noted on the physical aspects of care or the alleviation of pain, symptoms, or psychological distress. Families were only slightly more satisfied, although they were significantly less anxious than their conventional care counterparts. However, some hospice patients were cared for in general wards when hospice beds were full and hence were exposed to the conditions of the 'hospital group'. This may have led to a 'dilution of effect'.

Multi-site study on in-patient hospice care

Relatively few comparative studies in North America have examined in-patient hospice care compared to community-based hospice care and therefore no firm conclusions can be drawn. The New York Hospice Program focused on retrospective evaluations of patient and carer satisfaction four months after bereavement with the care provided across 12 hospice programs (Hannan and O'Donnell 1984). Comparisons were made between community-based programs, and two types of hospital-based programs: scattered beds and autonomous units. Equally high levels of satisfaction were reported by informal carers for services across the three settings. Estimations of patient satisfaction exceeded 90% for specific services provided across all settings, although satisfaction with care was higher for hospital-based programs than for community-based programs.

Non-comparative studies on in-patient hospice care

Non-comparative studies on views on in-patient hospice care have highlighted some of the perceived advantages from patient and informal carer perspectives. Perceived beneficial aspects of hospice care have included the homelike atmosphere, relaxed visiting hours and attention given to patients' families (Kellar *et al.* 1996). The importance placed on nursing care has been highlighted as a key aspect of hospice care in several studies (Harrison 1995, Kellar *et al.* 1996). Godkin *et al.* (1983) found that carers rated hospice care significantly higher than previously experienced forms of care, as they believed it facilitated better coping and emotional preparation for death.

Home care in North America: satisfaction and opinions

Comparative studies of various types of home care

Comparative studies on home care in North America have reaped contrary results with regard to satisfaction with multidisciplinary home care compared to ordinary home care (Hughes *et al.* 1992, Zimmer *et al.* 1985). A randomized controlled trial examining patient and carer satisfaction with a multidisciplinary primary home care team found significantly higher levels for this type of care compared to the control at 3 monthly follow-up periods over a 6 month period (Zimmer *et al.* 1985). Patients in the intervention group had fewer hospitalizations, nursing home visits, and out-patient visits. Care-giver satisfaction was associated with physician availability, competence, personal qualities, and treatment effects to a lesser extent. Another randomized controlled trial of hospital-based home care for patients found that significantly higher levels of satisfaction were expressed by patients and carers in the experimental group at 1 month into the care program but no significant differences were found at 6 months (Hughes *et al.* 1992). At the 6 month follow-up period, the sample size was substantially reduced owing to attrition, which may have influenced the outcome.

A retrospective interview survey of views on community-based hospice care of 47 bereaved care-givers before, during, and after terminal care in four community-based hospice programs found that satisfaction was generally high with regard to all hospice services (Foster 1987). Carers were more satisfied with services in areas where they held high expectations, had particular needs, or were well-informed by hospice staff (Foster 1987).

Few comparisons have been made with regard to satisfaction between specialist outreach home care and institutional care, which makes firm conclusions difficult to draw. A retrospective study by McCusker (1985) indicated that although home carers reported more problems and were less satisfied with the availability of care compared to those in the institutional group, they still expressed a preference for home care over institutional care.

Areas of concern with regard to home care

Although it is notable that satisfaction with most home care services is generally high (Zimmer *et al.* 1985, Goldstone 1992, Hughes *et al.* 1992), areas of concern have been highlighted in some studies. Amongst informal care-givers concerns have included inadequate sleep while caring for the patient during his or her last month of life, as well as the need for more overnight help and access to a respite service (Bramwell *et al.* 1995). McCusker (1985) found that ordinary home care users' concerns focused on the physical care of their patients, including inadequate pain control and the negative impact of a lack of respite care and distressing symptoms on the family. Other research has indicated that carers were not aware of the full range of services offered by community hospice services, including financial assistance, legal assistance, education, bereavement support, and counselling (Foster 1987).

Conclusion

Given the variety of ways in which satisfaction and consumer opinions can be measured, assessed and interpreted, comparing results across studies is inherently difficult. Researchers may focus on different aspects of care within the same model of palliative care and may examine patients for different lengths of time, or at different stages of their illness. It is therefore difficult to draw firm conclusions from the evidence.

Studies on consumer opinion in North America with regard to home care and in-patient and out-patient hospice care have reaped inconsistent results. Focusing on specific areas where consumers believe improvements are necessary and where benefits have occurred is slightly more fruitful.

Slightly clearer results have emerged from research in the UK with regard to consumer opinion on various models of palliative care.

Table 6.2 Comparative studies of patient /lay carer opinions or satisfaction with various types of palliative care in North America

Authors	Study design(s)	Intervention	Subjects[a]	Outcome measures	Results	Conclusions	Comments
Hughes et al. (1992)	Randomized control trial Diary study Interview survey Questionnaire survey	Randomized trial of the cost-effectiveness of hospital-based home care for the terminally ill, comparing traditional home care services with hospital based home care	Random sample of mainly terminally ill cancer patients with life expectancy of less than 6 months, with an informal care-giver. Total no: 171 Conventional home care (n = 85) Hospital-based home care (n = 86)	Patient and carer satisfaction and morale Psychological status Comparisons made at referral, 1 month, and 6 months.	Patients and carers in the hospital based home care group expressed significantly higher levels of satisfaction with care, compared to the control group at 1 month into care program (patient $p < 0.02$, care-giver $p < 0.005$) Patients and care-givers in the hospital-based care group reported higher levels of satisfaction with care compared to control group at 6 months but this was not significantly different possibly owing to reduced sample size	Hospital-based home care was regarded highly by both carers and patients	Strengths: RCT; no significant differences between groups at referral Weakness: Attrition; small sample size at follow-up
Foster et al. (1987)	Retrospective interview survey	Families' views on hospice care: on referral, compared to during care, compared to 3–6 months after bereavement	Family care-givers of patients who had died of cancer Total no: 47	Carer satisfaction	Primary care-givers expected on referral to receive: emotional support whilst caring for patient, respite care and symptom control from hospice care Primary care-givers were 'not sure' or 'did not expect' a range of services from hospices including financial assistance, legal and financial advice,	Primary care-givers were generally satisfied with all aspects of hospice care and expressed a preference for direct medical and emotional support services	Weakness: Retrospective views

Greer *et al.* (1986)	Interview survey	Comparison of conventional care with hospice care as part of the National Hospice Study. Comparisons were fortnightly until death of patient	Terminal cancer patients, with a primary care person 21 or older Total no: 1754 Hospice home care (*n* = 833) Hospital-based hospice (*n* = 624) Conventional cancer care (*n* = 297)	Carer satisfaction Costs Patient satisfaction	education, support after death of patient, counselling, and help with transport. Primary care-givers felt well informed about roles of hospice staff, how to reach them and where to find equipment, but less well informed about a range of issues such as symptom control and medical condition of patient Primary care-givers were 'mostly' to 'very much' satisfied with all hospice services and appeared to be a little more satisfied with those areas where they held high expectations and where they were well informed
					No significantly differences observed in patient's levels of satisfaction, which were high in all settings Hospital based and hospice care primary carer persons (PCP) reported higher satisfaction with patient care both before and after death, compared to PCPs of patients in conventional care PCPs of patients who received hospice care in either setting (hospital or home) were more satisfied with patients' place of death than PCPs of patients who	as opposed to spiritual and social-environment services. Terminally ill cancer patients were equally satisfied with hospital based hospice care, home care hospice and conventional care. Families of hospice patients were more satisfied with the place of patients' death compared

Table 6.2 (contd)

Authors	Study design(s)	Intervention	Subjects[a]	Outcome measures	Results	Conclusions	Comments
					received conventional care PCPs of both hospice home care patients and conventional care patients more likely to report that patient was able to remain at home as long as he/she wanted	to families of patients in the conventional care group	
Zimmer et al. (1985)	Randomized controlled trial Questionnaire survey	RCT of multi-disciplinary primary home healthcare team, compared to non-specialized home care).	Random sample of homebound, chronically or terminally ill elderly patients, dying of cancer, with a prognosis of less than 3 months. Total no: 158 at baseline only: home care group ($n = 82$) control group ($n = 76$)	Carer and patient satisfaction Health care utilization Mortality Psychological status	No significant differences between satisfaction levels at baseline, at 3 months and at 6 months for patients in both groups. Both indicated a trend towards greater satisfaction over time. Family care-givers in specialized home care team group showed significantly higher levels of satisfaction with care at 3 months and 6 months compared to the control group. Family care-givers' high levels of satisfaction in home care team associated with physician availability, competence, personal qualities, (and also treatment effects but to a lesser extent). Patients in the home care group	Informal family care-givers expressed significantly higher satisfaction with specialized home care team than control group for their care Associated with increased healthcare utilization and cost reduction.	

Study	Method	Aim	Sample	Measures	Results	Comments
McCusker *et al.* (1985)	Interview survey	Comparison of satisfaction with 'home care' compared to 'institutional care' during last 6 months of life. Interviews were carried out every 2 months until death, and with relatives 3–4 weeks after bereavement	Male and female terminally ill cancer patients. Total no: 122 patients (also 96 relatives interviewed and 122 physicians): Home care group (*n* = 54) Institutional group (*n* = 68)	Carer satisfaction Functional status Morbidity Patient/carer/professional's opinion	had fewer hospitalizations, nursing home admissions and out-patient visits than controls and used more in home services. Overall cost was lower than controls (but not significant). Most examples of satisfaction for both home and hospital care focused on qualities of specific health professionals (not treatments etc.). Almost one fifth of examples of dissatisfaction or both types of care concerned communication particularly with physicians. Relatives of patients who spent some of their last 6 months at home mentioned problems with physical care, patient experiencing distressing psychological symptoms, and negative impact of caring for patient at home on family. Relatives of home care group less satisfied with availability of care and reported that the patients experienced more pain compared to those in the institutional group. Relatives in the home care group reported a preference for home care	Relatives of patients who had used home care services were less satisfied with availability of care, reported inadequate pain control in patients and need for more respite care. In spite of these concerns, most relatives preferred home care than any other type of care. Strengths: 72% response rate for interviews of surviving relatives, 92% responses rate for interviews of physicians. 'Validity checks' were carried out 3–4 weeks after interview

Table 6.2 (contd)

Authors	Study design(s)	Intervention	Subjects[a]	Outcome measures	Results	Conclusions	Comments
Hannan and O'Donnell (1984)	Interview survey Questionnaire survey	Evaluation of the New York State Hospice Demonstration Program. Care in community based hospice vs. hospital-based hospice with 'scattered beds', vs. hospital-based hospice in an 'autonomous unit'	Patients receiving hospice care Total no: 350 primary care persons interviewed about 236 patients: Community-based hospice (n = 148) Hospital-based hospice scattered beds(n = 43) Hospital-based hospice autonomous unit (n = 159)	Patient and carer satisfaction Costs Impact of volunteers on care Utilization of care	PCPs estimations of patient satisfaction with specific services indicated overall satisfaction levels greater than 90% across all 3 models. PCP's views on patient's emotional and physical quality of life were mixed. PCP's estimations of patient's satisfaction with hospital care indicated significantly differences among 3 models of care – lower ratings for community-based care group. All PCPs found bereavement services either v. helpful or helpful.	High levels of satisfaction were associated with the provision of services, emotional support and bereavement services provided to the PCP Satisfaction with hospital care in hospital-based programmes was higher than for hospital care for community-based programmes, which may indicate that they have greater difficulty in incorporating in-patient components of programme	Weakness: Few details of patients given

| Kane *et al.* (1984) | RCT Interview survey | Comparison of hospice care with conventional care during last weeks/ months of life | Mainly male, terminally ill cancer patients with a prognosis of 2 weeks to 6 months. Total no: 247: Hospice group (*n* = 137) Control group (*n* = 110) | Patient and carer satisfaction Costs Functional status Length of stay Pain control Mortality Symptom control | No significant differences between groups on measures of pain, activities of daily living, symptoms or affect. Hospice patients more satisfied with the 'interpersonal care' compared to conventional care patients ($p < 0.01$) Family care-givers in hospice group were more satisfied and less anxious than those in conventional care group ($p < 0.05$) | Although hospice care was not more beneficial than conventional care in pain, symptom relief or alleviation of psychological distress, the higher levels of satisfaction shown by hospice patients and their families indicated an appreciation of other 'qualitative aspects' of hospice care |

Satisfaction with in-patient hospice care, home hospice care, and specialist outreach teams was generally high. Also, there was evidence to suggest that patients prefer to die at home, although their wishes are not always borne out in practice. Hospital and community care received a greater number of spontaneous criticisms and they were more wide ranging than the criticisms of hospice care, although it is notable that these were the views of a sizeable minority rather than the majority. In comparative terms, it is more difficult to determine which types of institutional, in-patient care are preferred. Indeed, since several comparative studies have involved comparisons of care provided by St Christopher's Hospice with other local institutions, it is difficult to rule out the potential influence of this pioneering centre on the quality and standards of palliative care provided in these institutions which are geographically close.

A key issue raised by comparative studies involving hospital care is the importance of considering the differential experiences of consumers dying from different diseases. Clearly more research is needed in this area, especially given the general movement towards enabling more non-cancer patients, especially people dying of HIV/AIDS, to receive better quality care based on palliative care principles.

Question 7

Impact on quality of life

CHRIS SALISBURY

What is the impact of different models of care on patients' quality of life, psychological well-being or motivation?

Methodology

For this chapter we have sought to identify all experimental and descriptive studies which evaluated a model of palliative care, and used quality of life as an outcome measure. The term 'quality of life' was interpreted broadly, to include not only formal measures which purport to assess quality of life as such but also measures of pain control, symptom control, or general well-being.

A large number of papers were identified which described the development of scales or research instruments to assess quality of life. These papers were excluded unless they included the use of the instrument to assess a model of care. However, reviews of approaches to the assessment of quality of life which included reviews of assessment tools were included. Studies which measured the impact of palliative care on the quality of life or bereavement process in relatives or carers were also excluded. Research which addressed the quality of life of cancer patients who were not necessarily terminally ill were not included unless a specific reference to terminally ill patients was included within the study.

What is quality of life, and how can it be measured?

Defining the concept

The concept of quality of life is hard to define, which makes its use as an outcome measure problematic. However, some assessment of the patient's well-being is clearly central to the evaluation of alternative models of palliative care. The problems of defining and measuring quality of life in the context of palliative care are of several types.

First, it is unclear which aspects of life should be assessed (McMillan 1996). One approach to the problem has been to ask people which aspects of their life are important to them in determining its quality. This approach has been used in the development of most assessment instruments for research. A number of reviews have been published on the assessment of quality of life in palliative care, and on the range of available assessment tools (de Haes and van Knippenberg 1985, Clark and Fallowfield 1986, Mor and Masterson-Allen 1987, Maguire and Selby 1989, Ahmedzai 1990, Aaronson 1991, Bullinger 1992, Goddard 1993, Finlay and Dunlop 1994, Cella 1995, Johnston and Abraham 1995, Fowlie and Berkeley 1987). These reviews suggest that quality of life is multidimensional, and instruments need to assess a number of constructs: symptom control, psychological well-being, social support, functional status, economic well-being, spiritual well-being, control over life, meeting life goals, and sexuality (Keay *et al.* 1994, McMillan and Mahon 1994a). McMillan and Mahon suggest that these issues can be summarized within four domains: physical/functional, social, psychological/spiritual, and economic (McMillan and Mahon 1994b, McMillan 1996). Several authors have shown that relief from pain is a major determinant of an individual's perception of quality of life (Ferrell *et al.* 1991).

Different assessment tools may not be comparable

The difficulty of defining quality of life raises the related problem that we cannot assume different research assessment tools are measuring the same thing. As a response to the large number of issues that people identify as important to quality of life, most assessment instruments are multidimensional, and combine scores across a number of scales. However, different assessment tools may measure a different range of aspects of quality of life and weight them differently. For example, the widely used Karnofsky scale is a measure of functional performance, and has only a low correlation with the more broadly based Sendera quality of life index (McMillan and Mahon 1994a).

Multidimensional scales which produce a global quality of life score may give an artificial precision to what is a diffuse and subjective concept. They may also mask important differences between patients, and between different models of care. For example, patients may rate hospice care as superior in some ways, but inferior in others (Goddard 1993), and this may be lost within a multidimensional scale. Such distinctions require the use of separate assessment tools, validated for the relevant patient population, which reliably and independently assess the relevant aims of the palliative care service in the study.

Subjective nature of quality of life

Although studies of people in general help to identify issues which are important to most people, the concept of quality of life is enormously subjective (Cella 1995). Any one individual may have values and priorities which are different from those of the group. This is particularly important in the context of palliative care, which places respect for an individual's autonomy and choices as a core value. Many quality of life measures have been validated for use with cancer patients rather than those who are terminally ill. The issues which are important to terminally ill patients may well be different, and may even change in the same individual as they approach death (Cohen and Mount 1992).

Recent studies of quality of life in palliative care have therefore focused on existential issues such as quality of personal meaning and purpose, which have been shown to be particularly important to dying patients (Cohen and Mount 1992, Viney *et al.* 1994, Cohen *et al.* 1996). One approach has been to develop assessment tools which allow patients to nominate areas of life that are important to them, such as SEIQoL (Hickey *et al.* 1996). These issues raise difficulties in establishing the reliability of quality of life measures in palliative care. The usual tests of inter-rater reliability and test–retest reliability are of no value for a subjective measure which is known to change rapidly (de Haes and van Knippenberg 1985).

Importance of using tools which reflect the aims

If quality of life measures are used to evaluate models of palliative care it is important to define the improvement that the palliative care service is seeking to achieve, as this will determine the appropriate measurement model (Viney *et al.* 1994). Degner *et al.* (1987) have emphasized the importance of having an underlying theory of coping in order to make meaningful evaluations. If the aim of a hospice is to help people come to terms with death, for example, then existing quality of life measures may not be meaningful or useful as they may not assess this. If inappropriate assessment tools are used, genuine improvements in care may not be detected (Wallston *et al.* 1988). The widely quoted National Hospice Study (Greer and Mor 1986, Greer *et al.* 1986) used the Spitzer Quality of Life Index. This decision was criticized before the study began because the Spitzer index does not reflect the existential concepts of meaning and integration which are important aims of hospices (Mount and Scott 1983).

Quality of life may change rapidly

Quality of life may vary considerably during the palliative care of a patient. Morris *et al.* (1986b) carried out a secondary analysis of quality of life data from the National Hospice Study (Greer and Mor 1986, Greer *et al.* 1986) and from a sample of terminally ill patients in Montreal. They showed that quality of life declined slowly, with accelerated deterioration in the final 3 weeks of life. Patient experience of pain was highly variable, and did not follow the same pattern as other quality of life measures: they therefore recommended that pain should be measured separately. Ventafridda *et al.* (1990) also showed that pain control did not correlate with other measures of quality of life. In a further study Morris and Sherwood (1987) showed that a similar rapid decline in quality of life in the final week of life occurred in settings other than hospices, but that the results were variable with a substantial minority of terminal patients retaining a good quality of life almost until death. This generally rapid but variable process of decline makes comparative studies across different settings and models of organization very difficult, unless patients are very carefully matched by time before death.

In practice, quality of life is often not defined by authors and varies from study to study (de Haes and van Knippenberg 1985). It may refer to a global evaluation or a combination of different domains, which may be differently weighted in different measurement tools, making comparison between studies difficult. In some cases studies have used 'home-grown' assessments or adaptations of existing instruments, with unknown reliability and validity.

Can care-givers act as proxies in quality of life assessments?

Patients who are terminally ill may not be able to complete complex research instruments, or it may be felt too intrusive to ask them to do so. The difficulties of obtaining quality of life assessments directly from patients have led several authors to use relatives, care-givers, or health professionals as proxies to assess patients' quality of life. The assumption that other people can reliably make assessments is assumed, for example, in Parkes' much quoted studies (Parkes 1980, Parkes and Parkes 1984).

Several authors have tested this assumption. Most studies have shown that neither care-givers nor staff are reliable proxies for the quality of life experienced by patients (Slevin *et al.* 1988, Higginson *et al.* 1990, Higginson *et al.* 1994a, McMillan and Mahon 1994a, McMillan and Mahon 1994b, McMillan 1996). Slevin *et al.* (1988) showed poor correlation between patients and doctors on a number of quality of life measures, with wide variability between different doctors' assessments of the same patient. Several studies have shown that care-givers rate patients' quality of life as significantly worse than patients do themselves (Cartwright and Seale 1990, Higginson *et al.* 1990, McMillan and Mahon 1994a,b). Higginson *et al.* (1990) showed that bereaved family members rated symptom control, pain control, and anxiety as worse than did the patients, but family members were more satisfied than patients with the support services. In a further study Higginson *et al.* (1994a) showed that there was poor agreement between staff and bereaved family members about the quality of symptom control which had been experienced by patients. McMillan (1996) studied the quality of life of patients with cancer receiving hospice care. She showed a moderate correlation between patients and care-giver reports for patients with a high quality of life, but the correlation declined as patient's quality of life deteriorated.

By contrast, a few studies have suggested that staff or patients may be reasonably reliable proxies. One was a very small study of only 23 patients (Curtis and Fernsler 1989). The second (Higginson and McCarthy 1993) compared the assessments of patients, their families, and staff as part of the validation of a new quality of life schedule. scores by palliative care team member correlated moderately well with patients' assessments, and better than family members' assessments. Staff identified more problems than did patients, except in the area of pain control. A similar study also showed that staff, patients, and relatives provided similar scores using the Support Team Assessment Schedule (Butters *et al.* 1993).

However, the overall weight of evidence suggests that studies which rely on care-giver or staff assessments of patients' quality of life should be accorded less weight than those that used patients' own assessments.

Impact of models of palliative care on patients' quality of life

A number of papers were identified and reviewed which described the quality of life, pain control, or symptom control of terminally ill patients in a number of different settings, but with no comparisons. This included longitudinal studies which showed the change in individual patients' quality of life during a program of care, but without a control group it is not possible to relate the model of care to the changes in the patients' status. Brief details of these non-comparative studies are shown in Table 7.1, but relatively little weight is given to them in the conclusions.

Comparative studies of palliative care with quality of life or symptom control as an outcome

Comparative studies are shown in more detail in Table 7.2. This includes any study of terminally ill patients which seeks to compare the quality of life of patients under different models of care. The table describes research using many different methodologies. Few studies used randomized control groups; several were evaluations of the quality of life of patients before and after the institution of a new programme of care. Of those studies which did have control groups most were retrospective, with matched rather than randomly allocated control groups. There is considerable potential for con-founding variables in terms of prognosis, type and stage of disease, and patient characteristics. However well the matching was carried out, it is never possible to exclude confounding factors which were not anticipated. Selection bias is likely with different forms of care attracting different types of patients.

It is acknowledged that some methodologies are less prone to bias than others, and the type of design, the strength and weakness of the study, and the generalizability of the results all need to be considered when drawing conclusions.

Summary of key research papers

Studies from the USA and Europe

The largest and most rigorously conducted studies to evaluate the impact of alternative models of palliative care on quality of life are the National Hospice Study and the UCLA hospice evaluation study, both carried out in the US during the early 1980s. The National Hospice Study (Greer *et al.* 1983, Aiken 1986, Greer *et al.* 1986, Greer and Mor 1986, Morris *et al.* 1986a, Wallston *et al.* 1988) involved over 1700 patients, and compared patients receiving home-based hospice care, hospital in-patient hospice care, and conventional care. This was an observational study, based on 40 hospices and 14 conventional care sites. Patients were selected for follow-up according to cancer site, presence of a primary care-giver, functional performance status, and willingness to take part. The conventional care sites were selected not to represent typical conventional care, but as examples of the best available conventional care. Multivariate statistical analysis was carried out to determine differences between the group of patients on a wide range of outcomes (including quality of life), after adjustment for the effects of differences in the patient populations.

There was no evidence from the National Hospice Study that patients' quality of life was affected by care in a hospital-based hospice, a home-based hospice, or a conventional care site. Hospital-based hospice patients had slightly better pain control and greater use of analgesics.

The lack of impact on quality of life was not, however, interpreted as a negative result. The motivation for the study was a concern that hospices, with a philosophy of reducing medical intervention, might actually deprive patients of essential medical care and lead to a lower quality of life. The authors' conclusion was that hospice care

Table 7.1 Impact of models of palliative care on quality of life or symptom control: non-comparative descriptive studies

Author	Country	Disease	Details of study	Results	Key conclusions	Comments
Barzelai (1981)	USA	Cancer	Interview survey of care-givers of patients cared for by home care hospice	82% of patients experienced pain relief, 88% relief of other symptoms	Respondents reported that hospice was helpful in reducing prevalence of pain, physical symptoms and anxiety	Good response rate (20/24). Small study, unsophisticated questionnaire, no controls. Care-givers' assessment as proxies, retrospectively
Wilkes (1984)	UK	Mixed	Descriptive study of patients dying in hospital or at home	Many uncontrolled symptoms. Many carers critical of general practitioners and hospital, but much praise for nursing staff. A quarter of caring relatives aged over 70. Difficulties of relatives more often a cause for admission than those of patient	Very varied quality of care provided both in primary care and in hospitals as perceived by patients. Poor symptom control in many patients	Very subjective assessments, which varied considerably between relatives, doctors and nurses. Limited data reported, percentages without base numbers
Higginson and McCarthy (1989)	UK	Cancer	Description of symptoms at referral and during care by support team	Pain was main symptom in 35/86 patients at referral, pain scores improved within 1 week of care, and improved further towards death. Dyspnoea scores did not improve with team support. Overall symptom scores improved after referral	Pain is main reason for referral to palliative care support team, and symptoms can be improved with care	Without control group is impossible to ascribe improvement to the support team (although this is likely): authors wisely do not make this claim.
Ventafridda et al. (1990)	Italy	Cancer	Changes in QoL assessment during palliative care	During treatment, decreased proportion of patients reported pain, weakness, functional	Pain is important determinant of suffering, but not	Use of results from patients at different stages since onset of

			program (home, out-patients, in-patients, combined results)	impairment or psychological distress. Global sense of 'feeling well' improved. Lack of pain correlated most strongly with 'feeling well'. Pain control did not correlate with other measures of QoL, whereas psychological and functional measures did correlate with each other	necessarily representative of other domains of QoL	palliative care makes analysis hard to interpret
Woodruff et al. (1991)	Australia	Mixed	Description of multidisciplinary care team to advise about palliative care in hospital	Pain control was problem in 40% of patients, other physical symptoms important in 31%. Intensive counselling for psychological problems provided in 70%. 72% required liaison with domiciliary care services	Multidisciplinary nature of team is crucial to its success in achieving aims of providing care, symptom control, communication with other agencies	Straightforward retrospective study from records, no comparisons made
Miller and Walsh (1991)	USA	Cancer	Range of psychosocial problems at presentation of patients referred to palliative care	63% anxious, 54% sad/depressed. 54% had only one care-giver	Terminal care patients have multiple social and psychological problems, and many do not have sufficient help at home to look after them	No validation or rigour in research instrument. Descriptive only, no control. Very limited useful data presented
Butters et al. (1992)	UK	HIV / AIDS	Impact of 2 home care teams on QoL	Between referral and death, symptom control ratings improved ($p < 0.01$) as did patient anxiety ($p < 0.0001$), and pain control ($p < 0.0001$), and practical aid	Symptom control (weakness, diarrhoea, muscle wasting, memory loss, visual	Ratings based on carer perceptions, but previous studies have found high rate of inter-rater reliability between

Table 7.1 (contd)

Author	Country	Disease	Details of study	Results	Key conclusions	Comments
				($p < 0.001$). Symptom control was commonly a severe problem at referral and remained a serious problem throughout care, whereas patient anxiety and pain control although initially severe improved more substantially	problems, dyspnoea) proved most difficult for teams to achieve especially in last week of care	patient and carer on STAS ratings
Higginson et al. (1992b)	UK	Cancer	STAS results for patients seen by two palliative support teams	Out of 17 items, all but 2 (family anxiety and spiritual) improved during care. 16% of patients did not improve. Symptom control remained problematic until death.	Demonstrates value of measuring key indicators using measure designed to reflect aims of palliative care	Well-designed study. Impossible to attribute improvements to the support team in an observational study (although this seems likely)
O'Brien et al. (1992)	UK	MND	Description of management of patients from case notes	Patients very dependent: need for nursing care was main reason for referral. Most patients deteriorated suddenly, then died within 24 hours	MND patients have problems which are appropriately managed in a hospice	Uncontrolled descriptive study
Mercadante et al. (1992)	Italy	Cancer	Observational study of home palliative care team—results as team expanded	At point of referral, few patients had received opioids, and pain control ineffective in 60–75% of cases. With home care, pain control was achieved in 80–95% of cases	Possible to control symptoms, especially pain, in terminal care using home care	Limited study, only describes pain. Main outcomes (pain) not assessed rigorously. An uncontrolled study, so patients'

Study	Country	Patients	Aim	Findings	Conclusion	Critique
Maddocks et al. (1994)	Australia	Leukaemia and others	Characteristics of patients and events surrounding death for patients with leukaemia by comparison with other deaths	More than half leukaemia patients needed more than one admission in final month of life. Few leukaemia patients referred to palliative care team, all died in hospital. Leukaemia patients experienced similar symptom profile to patients dying of colorectal cancer	Since most leukaemia patients will die in hospital, need palliative care support in hospital as well as at home and hospice	Very small study with insufficient power to generalize robust conclusions
McMillan and Mahon (1994a)	USA	Mixed	Quality of life of hospice patients on admission and week 3, comparison of patients and care-givers assessments	No significant differences in Sendara index from weeks 0–3, half patients experienced significant improvement, others deteriorated. Only weak correlation (r = 0.45 week 0, 0.39 week 3) between patient and carer assessments. Only weak correlation (r = 0.25) between Sendara and Karnofsky scores	Lack of deterioration in QoL over 3 weeks may indicate success of hospice care for some people	Only 67/460 patients included in study, others too ill, so very selected population, and only 31/67 survived to complete a score after 3 weeks. Care-givers not a reliable proxy as assessors of patients' QoL.
Hinton (1994a)	UK	Cancer	Assessment of problems experienced by patients and relatives supported by home hospice care	Tolerable physical symptoms volunteered by 63%. 50% reached positive acceptance of dying, 11% of patients were distressed. Preference for home care fell steadily from 100% to 54% for patients and 45% for relatives. Patients and relatives satisfied with care provided at home	Home care is acceptable for most people, most of the time, but significant minorities need in-patient care towards very end of life	Very subjective assessments made by professional associated with the hospice service concerned, so not unbiased. Detailed qualitative assessments, based on weekly or fortnightly interviews

responses likely to reflect efforts made on their behalf.

Table 7.1 (contd)

Author	Country	Disease	Details of study	Results	Key conclusions	Comments
Addington-Hall *et al.* (1995)	UK	Stroke	Symptom control in last year of life based on analysis of data from Regional study of Care for the Dying	More than half patients had experienced inadequately controlled pain, also confusion, low mood, urinary incontinence. One quarter to one fifth of relatives dissatisfied with aspects of hospital in patient care. One third felt hospital doctors too rushed, many unmet needs for information	Improvements needed in symptom control, provision of information, and education about principles of palliative care for those caring for stroke patients	Secondary analysis of retrospective study. Uncontrolled descriptive data. Rigorous and detailed data collection
Ellershaw *et al.* (1995)	UK	Cancer	Impact of hospital PCST	Within 4 days of PCST involvement there were statistically significantly improvements in pain control ($p < 0.001$), nausea ($p < 0.009$), insomnia ($p < 0.004$), and anorexia ($p < 0.001$), maintained at day 7 at which time relief of constipation was also achieved ($p < 0.02$)	A hospital palliative care team is effective at improving symptom control	Used a measure of demonstrable reliability and validity. Observational uncontrolled study, so impossible to confidently ascribe improvements to the care team
Talmi *et al.* (1995)	Israel	Cancer	Description from chart audit of characteristics of patients with head and neck cancer	32% of patients had difficult feeding, 22% had airway problems. Pain was severe in 60% of patients, light/moderate in 22%. 50% of patients died within 10 days of admission	Claims that these patients may receive better care in hospice than general hospital, although no data shown to support this	Descriptive study, no comparison with defined standards or control group. No detailed description of how outcomes, e.g. pain, were assessed.

Study	Country	Diagnosis	Study aim	Findings	Conclusion	Comments
Oliver (1996)	UK	MND	Hospice care of patients with MND	Weakness, dysphagia, dyspnoea and pain were main problems for these patients. Most required morphine. 48% died at home	Co-ordination of services needed to care for these patients at home	Description of only one hospice, no information about how representative these patients are
Jarvis *et al.* (1996)	Canada	Mixed	Impact of palliative care program on symptoms at admission and at 1 week; patient and carer satisfaction, use of resources, staff stress	Re QoL, only 34/84 patients assessed at both admission and 1 week. Mean symptom score improved for in-patients, those in consultation care, home support but not long-term care. Only significant for consultation care, because of small numbers. Improvements for consultation care patients in outlook, pain frequency, insomnia, appetite, bowel function	Overall symptom distress reduced, especially for consultation care patients	Very small numbers, so may not detect genuine differences. More than half of patients initially assessed died, and a 'large number' of patients were initially excluded, so selected sample
Courtens *et al.* (1996)	Netherlands	Cancer	Longitudinal study of changes in QoL after diagnosis.	QoL positively related to emotional support. Over time, size of social networks decreased	A relationship between QoL and social support, but does not indicate causality	Well conducted study. Only 51 patients
McMillan (1996)	USA	Cancer	Descriptive study of QoL of cancer patients receiving hospice care	Four factors identified: social/ spiritual; psychological/ emotional; physical/functional; financial. QoL scores were stable and reliable. Carers' reports of patients QoL were lower and only moderately correlated with patients own reports	QoL can be measured by a valid and reliable instrument. QoL is characterized by multidimensionality and subjectivity	Findings based on a non-random group of patients in only one setting

Table 7.2   Comparative studies to evaluate the impact of models of

Author	Country	Subjects	Study design	Comparison
Parkes (1978)	UK	Spouses of patients who had died of cancer in Lewisham or Bromley Total no. 276: 65 'home-centred' 100 'hospital centred'	interview survey, retrospective study	Patients who had received predominantly hospital or home-based terminal care
Parkes (1979)	UK	Surviving spouses of patients dying at St Christopher's hospice Total no. 89: 55 hospice 34 elsewhere	NRCT	Patients dying at St. Christopher's hospice vs. matched pairs dying at other hospitals
Hinton (1979)	UK	Cancer patients, prognosis <3 mths, married, not in serious physical distress. Total no: 80 (20 in each group; see 'comparison')	Observational study Interview survey	Comparison of mood and opinion of patients in in-patient hospice, foundation home, general hospital, out-patient hospice

palliative care on quality of life or symptom control

QoL measurement tools	Results	Key conclusions	Comments
Interviews of spouses	Patients dying at home had increase in pain towards death, those dying in hospital had decrease in pain. Patients in hospital more likely to be confused or confined to bed. More than 1/5 of patients experienced severe pain at death in both settings	Important deficiencies in care in both home and hospital. Terminal care at home associated with more pain than hospital care.	Interviews long after bereavement (mean 13 months). Uncontrolled study; different types of patients will have been treated in home and hospital. Arbitrary distinction between groups—'home' patients received some hospital care and vice versa
Semi-structured interviews	Patients well matched for age, sex, s.e. status, length of terminal period. Hospice patients had more severe pain before admission. Fewer hospice patients had severe pain (18% vs 48%) ($p < 0.05$). Fewer hospice patients were confined to bed ($p < 0.05$). No difference in conscious level or confusion. Fewer hospice patients suffered moderate/ severe distress ($p < 0.05$)	Hospice provides less pain and distress for terminally ill patients	Retrospective views of relatives (of doubtful use as proxies), long after the event. Interviews not blind, may have been biased. Spouses involved in 'community' of St Christopher's may have felt loyal to it. (Part II, not evaluated here, shows that spouses at hospices spent much more time there and got to know staff and other patients well.)
Scaled ratings completed by researcher from interviews with patient, spouse, senior nurse	Re QoL: Patients in in-patient hospice showed less depression ($p < 0.05$), anxiety ($p < 0.001$) and anger ($p < 0.01$) than in other settings	In-patient hospice generates least distress for patients, but good care possible in all settings studied	Assessments not blind, nor objective; very open to bias. Correlation with nurse and spouse assessment said to be good but Kappa is more appropriate test, and few details given. Concepts of depression, anxiety, anger not defined—better measures are available. Patients likely to have different characteristics in the four settings. More of a descriptive study than providing useful comparisons

Table 7.2 (contd)

Author	Country	Subjects	Study design	Comparison
Parkes (1980)	UK	Spouses of patients dying from cancer in 2 London boroughs 1. Total no: 102 (51 matched pairs) 2. Total no: 462 (23 pairs matched by age, sex, social class, duration of treatment, pain)	Interview survey	1. Patients visited by home care team vs. those not visited. 2. Patients dying in hospital previously cared for by hospice or not
Parkes and Parkes (1984)	UK	Surviving spouses of patients dying of cancer in 1977–79 Total no: 164: 42 hospice 122 hospitals	retrospective study Interview survey	Perceptions of spouses of hospice patients vs. other hospitals and vs. similar study 10 years earlier
Zimmer et al. (1984, 1985)	USA	Housebound chronically ill or terminally ill elderly Total no. 167: 85 home care 82 controls	RCT	Terminal and non-terminal groups receiving home care team, and controls
Kane et al. (1984, 1985a,b)	USA	Patients with terminal cancer admitted to veterans teaching hospital Total no: 247 137 hospice 110 controls	RCT	Hospice care vs. routine care

QoL measurement tools	Results	Key conclusions	Comments
Interviews with bereaved spouses	Re symptom control and QoL: no difference between patients visited by home care team and others in relief of pain, breathlessness, nausea or other symptoms. No difference in psychological symptoms. (several other aspects of care not examined here)	No difference in terms of perceived QoL between patients receiving or not receiving home care team	Based on bereaved spouses retrospective reports, long after the event (mean of 13 months later). No evidence whether spouses were reliable proxy. No validated instruments used, just interview data of spouses' recollections of symptom control
Semi-structured interviews and symptom scores	Patients suffered less pain in both settings than in 1967–69. Spouses reported less anxiety at both settings than in 1967–69 with fewer spouses or hospices reporting severe anxiety than elsewhere. Spouses more involved in care at hospice than at other hospitals	Improvements in all settings in terminal care from perspective of spouses may be attributed to educational impact of hospice	Few details of methodology and of selection of 'other hospitals'. Non-blind assessments. Difficult to know if patients were comparable in two groups despite attempt to compare matched pairs of patients
Date and place of death, patient and carer satisfaction questionnaire, PGC morale scale, Sickness Impact Profile, Utilization Diary	No differences in SIP profile (only measure relevant to QoL) either at 3 or 6 months	Home care team had no measurable impact on QoL	Well-designed study. Not all patients were terminally ill, so not necessarily entirely relevant
Anxiety scale from General Well-being Measure, CES-D depression scale, Involvement in care scale, Katz activity of daily living index, McGill Pain Scale, Physical environment scale, Satisfaction scale	No differences in length of survival, place of death, number of in-patient days, costs, number of invasive procedures, pain control, symptom control, ADL scores, depression. Hospice patients more satisfied with care ($p < 0.01$), and with involvement in care ($p < 0.01$) and their family care-givers expressed less anxiety ($p < 0.01$)	No differences between hospice and conventional care in effectiveness or cost, but patients preferred hospice care	Almost all male veteran patients, not representative of general population. Some contamination between groups, with control group staff probably influenced by hospice staff attitudes. Also hospice patients spent a third of their in-patient time in general medical wards. Outcome measures mostly adapted from other scales; reliability and validity of adapted versions unknown

Table 7.2   (contd)

Author	Country	Subjects[a]	Study design	Comparison
Greer et al. (1986), Greer and Mor (1986) (also see Morris et al. 1986a)	USA	Cancer patients with metastases aged >21 and with a primary care-giver, and (for conventional care patients only) requiring assistance in daily activities. Total no. 1754 624 Hospital based hospice (HB) 833 Home care hospice (HC) 297 Conventional care (CC)	NRCT	HB vs.HC vs. CC
Morris et al. (1986a)	USA	Patients with metastatic cancer, aged >21, with primary care-giver. Total no. 1754 624 HB 833 HC 297 CC	NRCT	Pain control in HB, HC, CC
Wallston et al. (1988)	USA	Subset of patients from national hospice study who died of cancer within 6 months of entering study and whose principal carer participated in a bereavement interview Total no. 880	NRCT	Comparison of quality of death across HB, HC, and CC Secondary analysis of data from National Hospice Study

[a] Subjects, total number and number in each group

QoL measurement tools	Results	Key conclusions	Comments
'Uniscale', assessments of primary care-giver, Composite pain index (modified from Spitzer), Composite symptom severity scale (modified from Melzach), Emotional QoL judged by PCP, HRCA index, Karnofsky performance status, Patient awareness judged by PCP, Social QoL (various)	Patients in either type of hospice had fewer intensive interventions. (eg. blood transfusions; intravenous therapy) No differences between groups on wide range of QoL indicators. HB patients had slightly less pain than HC or CC patients and greater prescription and consumption of analgesics. HB patients had fewer symptoms than HC or CC patients at 3 weeks before death	Hospice care provides alternative philosophy of care, a viable alternative, with no difference from conventional care in terms of effect on QoL	Sites not randomly selected, and each group (especially CC) is very varied. CC groups were selected as sites providing good quality care. May not be typical. Major differences in patient characteristics between groups, with CC patients younger, less functional ability. 20.6% of CC patients refused to participate compared with 3.3% of HC and 3.5% of HB patients. Many measures based on care-givers' perceptions which may not be reliable proxy
Composite symptom score adapted from Melzach pain index adapted from Spitzer QoL index.	Patient and care-giver reports of pain had correlation of 0.43. According to care-givers, 16% of patients were pain free in last weeks of life, proportion in persistent pain increased from 12% to 18% in final 4 weeks of life HB patients less likely to report persistent pain than HC or CC patients	HB patients may receive better pain control	Incomplete data is presented, in particular was improved pain control in HB patients also demonstrated in patients own accounts? How different were pain levels at outset of study in different settings? Major differences between characteristics of patients in 3 settings may not be wholly adjusted for by regression equations
'Quality of death' score	QoD scores lower for CC (mean 72.5) than HC (mean 80.4) and HB (mean 81.5) ($p < 0.03$) Effect remained after adjustment for confounders e.g. age, sex, extent of disease at diagnosis	Earlier QoL score insufficiently sensitive to capture issues of quality of death which are important to dying patients. Main differences between scores based on hospice patients being free of pain, and able to stay at home as long as wanted	Non-randomized trial: possible differences between patients in hospices and conventional care, not adjusted for Based on primary carers' perception of death—proxy may be unreliable, and biased by values derived from contact with hospice

Table 7.2   (contd)

Author	Country	Subjects	Study design	Comparison
Mor *et al.* (1988b)	USA	Male patients with cancer Total no. 442 229 day-hospital 213 in-patients	RCT Interview survey, cost–benefit analysis	Day hospital vs. in-patient cancer care while receiving cytotoxic chemotherapy
Ventafridda *et al.* (1989)	Italy	Terminal cancer patients aged 20–70 Total no. 60 (30 each group)	observational study	Comparison of 30 sequential patients cared for in hospital or by home care team
Seale (1991b)	UK	Closest relatives or other informants of random sample of deaths from cancer in people aged >15 1. Total no. 171 45 hospice 126 other cancer patients 2. Total no. 52 (26 matched pairs)	retrospective study, interview survey	1. Comparison of hospice and CC patients 2. Analysis of matched pairs

QoL measurement tools	Results	Key conclusions	Comments
Karnofsky performance status, McGill pain questionnaire, profile of mood states (POMS), Rand satisfaction with medical care scale, Spitzer QoL index, therapeutic response, WHO toxicity rating	No difference in therapeutic response, or treatment-related toxicity. No significant differences in number and severity of symptoms. Reported QoL, mood state and satisfaction with medical care was similar for patients in both groups at 20 and 60 days. Of 17% of ADH patients previously/subsequently treated in the hospital, 87% said they preferred ADH	Selected cancer patients currently receiving treatment in hospital can be treated on a day hospital basis with no negative effects on clinical or psychosocial status and with 25–30% savings in medical costs. Patients preferred to return home at night and this did not place a greater burden on patients and families	Well designed and conducted trial. Not specifically palliative care
Daily pain score—self judged, Spitzer QoL index	Cases well matched in age, sex, marital status; but home care patients better educated and different cancer sites. No differences between home and hospital care for pain or number of symptoms. After 2 weeks, home care patients had slightly better Karnofsky performance ($p = 0.01$), better QoL ($p = 0.001$). Patients more satisfied with sufficiency of care ($p = 0.037$). Home care cost less	Home care can provide qualitatively superior care than hospital because of functional and subjective improvements, rather than improvements in symptoms or pain control. Achieved at lower costs	May well be selection bias between patients choosing home or hospital care. Small numbers of patients, limited power. Statistical information to support conclusions is limited and incomplete, e.g. shows standard deviations when standard errors or confidence intervals more appropriate
Extensive interview	Hospice patients were younger, and less likely to have non-cancer diagnoses. Had more symptoms, and more functional restrictions. More religious, more likely to know they would die, less likely to have had operation in last year of life. Hospice patients had better relief from pain, more likely to have had room to themselves	Process of death for hospice patients clearly different from non-hospice patients, and differences valued by closest informants	Significant differences between types of people and severity of illness admitted to hospices and conventional care. Impossible to account fully for confounders—pairs matched only on sex and cancer site

Table 7.2   (contd)

Author	Country	Subjects	Study design	Comparison
Addington-Hall *et al.* (1992)	UK	Cancer patients with life expectancy < 1 year. Total no. 554 318 co-ordination group 236 controls	RCT Interview survey	Nurse co-ordinators plus routine services vs. routine services only
Hughes *et al.* (1992)	USA	Patients with prognosis < 6 mths, with a primary care-giver. Predominantly male veterans Total no. 171 85 control 86 intervention	RCT	Hospital based home care (HBHC), a multidisciplinary team managing care in and out of hospital vs. routine care, not involving HBHC at same or other hospital or hospice
Dessloch *et al.* (1992)	Germany	Terminally ill cancer patients 41 20 hospice, 21 hospital	Observational study	HBHC vs. hospital care

QoL measure-ment tools	Results	Key conclusions	Comments
Family Apgar scale, Hospital Anxiety and Depression scale, Interviews, Leeds depression and anxiety scale, SQLI	Co-ordinated group received more effective treatment for vomiting (OR 0.04 (0.02–0.79)) and constipation (OR 0.14 (0.04–0.51)).Co-ordinated group carers more likely to have seen chiropodist (OR 7.14(0.85–50.0)) and to contact specialist nurse in night-time emergency (OR 0.14 (0.02–1.17)) Carers less likely to feel angry at death of patient (OR 3.1 (1.15–8.3))	Few significant differences between group receiving co-ordinator and control. Maybe because nursing background of co-ordinators was inappro-priate to the role, or maybe co-ordination needed own budget to obtain services	Many comparisons, so a few symptom differences are likely due to chance. V. wide confidence interval (small numbers of patients remaining) means some genuine differences may have been undetected. High drop-out rate (63% (351/554)) because of deaths, refusals, moved away
Barthels self care index, Philadelphia Geriatric Centre Morale Scale, Satisfaction with care scale (Greer), Short Portable Mental Status questionnaire	98% of HBHC group received home visits, 52% of controls received some home healthcare No difference in func-tional self care status, cog-nitive status, morale, but improvement in patients satisfaction ($p = 0.04$ at 1 mth, 0.06 at 6 mths). Care-givers experienced more satisfaction with care at 1 mth ($p < 0.001$) but not at 6 mths; lower morale by 6 mths HBHC patients received more home nursing visits ($p = 0.001$) fewer out-patient visits ($p = 0.01$) and fewer days as in-patient (10 vs. 16 days $p = 0.03$)	HBHC improves access to home-based care with greater patient and carer satisfaction, at lower cost, with no impact on functional status	No measure of pain or symptom control. QoL assessments limited. No details of randomization No details of how much hospice care control group received
Semi-structured interview schedule	Patients matched by physical condition HBHC superior for perceived control over daily activities and caring routines, satisfaction with nursing, positive environ-ment. No difference in terms of social support and distress, coping with illness, physical well-being, satisfaction with medical care	Limited advantage of HBHC	Very small non-randomized sample. May well be selection bias. Unlikely to demonstrate any but very large differences; significance of differences reported is unknown. (Reviewed from abstract only)

Table 7.2   (contd)

Author	Country	Subjects	Study design	Comparison
Siegel *et al.* (1992)	USA	Patients with cancer of breast/ bowel/ lung, receiving out-patient chemotherapy, aged >21 Total no. 398 266 intervention group 132 control	RCT	Automated telephone contact to initiate social worker intervention for unmet needs
McWhinney *et al.* (1994)	Canada	Patients with metastatic cancer, aged over 18, prognosis < 2 months Total no. 146 randomized; only 76 completed trial	RCT	Home care team vs. control (to receive home care team after 1 month wait)
Viney *et al.* (1994)	Australia	Dying of cancer Total no. 183 62 small hospice 60 large hospice 61 hospital	Observational study. Interview survey, questionnaire survey	Patients in small hospice/ large hospice/ small general hospital

QoL measurement tools	Results	Key conclusions	Comments
Unmet needs identified by computer generated telephone survey	Fewer patients in experimental group reported unmet needs with heavy housekeeping, transportation to hospital, filling out forms, medical supervision and equipment. Differences not significant. 95/109 patients in experimental group had been contacted by social worker in response to survey and reported needs. Unclear how many in control group had any contact with social worker	Automated telephone generated survey follow-up is feasible, and may enable identification of unmet needs	Insufficient patient numbers to generate significant conclusions. Final assessment not apparently 'blind'. Unclear whether benefit should be ascribed to telephone follow-up or social work intervention, since 87% of experimental group needed social worker in response to survey
McGill pain questionnaire, Melzack nausea questionnaire, QoL—functional living index	Project abandoned. Only 146/307 patients were suitable, only 97 successfully followed up at 1 month, only 74 caregivers completed questionnaire	Problems of recruitment, attrition, exposure of control group to intervention, ethical problems of randomization, low compliance make RCTs very difficult in palliative care	Problems identified were partially caused by carrying out trial after the service had been operational for 18 months
Six scales representing psychological aspects of QoL	Patients in palliative care units expressed more positive feelings and less indirectly expressed anger, more anxiety about death and less general anxiety, than hospital patients. Those in smaller units showed more directly expressed anger and helplessness than those in larger palliative care units	Patients in specialized palliative care units differed from patients dying in a general hospital in terms of some psychological measures of QoL	Possibility of difference in patient groups in different units, not comparable Only some prior hypotheses supported: *post hoc* theories based on statistical associations are of doubtful validity unless confirmed elsewhere

Table 7.2   (contd)

Author	Country	Subjects	Study design	Comparison
McQuillan *et al.* (1996)	UK	All eligible patients with terminal HIV or cancer admitted to Department of Palliative Care Total no. 334 178 in 1991 146 in 1993	Before and after study	Introduction of palliative care support service (doctor and pharmacist)
Higginson and Hearn (1997)	UK and Ireland	Advanced cancer total no. 695 Effect on pain control reported for 358 patients in care >2 weeks 485 at home 173 in hospital or hospice	Before and after study	Assessment before and after referral to palliative care team

QoL measurement tools	Results	Key conclusions	Comments
Patient rating of pain and nausea (patient symptom score).	Pain score improved in 1993 compared to 1991. 22% of patients claimed their pain worsened in 1991 but only 15% in 1993. (Not statistically significant.) There were trends towards improvement for nausea, vomiting, constipation and sore mouth (also not significant)	Prescribing and symptom control, particularly in respect to pain, improved following the introduction of palliative care services	Before and after trial—other changes apart from support team will have occurred Assessors of symptom control were involved in the project so may be biased. Trends to improvement not significant
Karnofsky Performance Index; pain item from STAS	Significant reduction in pain after 2 weeks of specialist care ($p < 0.0001$), proportion in severe/overwhelming pain reduced from 14% to 4%. No relationship between pain score and Karnofsky score. Change in Karnofsky score after 2 weeks not reported.	Prevalence of pain in advanced cancer patients in community as high as in hospital. Multidisciplinary palliative care teams effective at alleviating pain. Karnofsky score not a good measure of effect of pain on patient	Limitations of before and after design. Variety of models of care assessed together (some community based, some hospital-based, working in different healthcare systems in England and Ireland) Assessment of pain by key team worker was non-blind, likely to be prone to bias Multicentre study which does reflect the full range of cancer patients usually treated by palliative care—good generalizability

RCT, randomized controlled trial

provides an acceptable alternative to conventional care, at no greater cost, and with greater patient satisfaction (Aiken 1986).

The impact of hospice on the cost of care and the quality of life of terminal patients is complex. There appear to be few robust patient quality of life advantages associated with hospice, and although the home care model reduces costs the hospital-based model may not. The appropriate policy response to those results depends on the value we place upon free choice in our society. Since hospice apparently has no negative effects and it costs no more (it may be both more effective and less costly in certain circumstances), from a social policy perspective it is a viable alternative for terminal care. (Greer and Mor 1986)

The UCLA study was the only randomized controlled trial to evaluate in-patient hospice care (Wales *et al.* 1983, Kane *et al.* 1984, 1985a,b, Kane 1986). Terminally ill cancer patients at a veterans' administration hospital were randomly assigned to receive hospice care or conventional care. Hospice care was provided in a special in-patient unit (but see criticisms below) or at home; conventional care consisted of the usual plan of treatment from the patients' named doctors at home and in general hospital wards. This study provided very similar results to the National Hospice Study. No differences were found between patients receiving hospice or conventional care in terms of quality of life, pain control, symptom control, or a range of other variables. Hospice patients expressed more satisfaction with care, and with their involvement in care, and less anxiety.

Both the National Hospice Study and the UCLA study are open to a number of criticisms which are detailed in Table 7.2 and have been discussed in published reviews (Mor and Masterson-Allen 1987, Broadfield 1988, Higginson and McCarthy 1989, Seale 1989, Goddard 1993, Johnston and Abraham 1995).

A randomized controlled trial of a home-based care team in US patients who were chronically or terminally ill was described by Zimmer *et al.* (1985). This well-designed study may not be entirely relevant to the UK provision of palliative care because it was not specifically concerned with palliative care, and because of the different healthcare system. This study failed to demonstrate any effect of the home care team on quality of life, although positive results were shown in other ways. Hughes *et al.* (1992) carried out a randomized controlled trial of home-based hospice care but with an emphasis on studying cost-effectiveness. Quality of life measures were limited, but no differences were seen between groups in terms of activities of daily living or cognitive functioning. An Italian non-randomized comparison of patients' home-based palliative care with conventional care also showed only limited effect of the home care programme on quality of life issues. In this study the home care patients achieving slightly better functional status but no improvements in pain or symptom control (Ventafridda *et al.* 1989).

UK studies

Several papers have described the evaluation of palliative care through the analysis of matched pairs of patients. Seale (1991b) interviewed 171 relatives of patients who had died in hospice or conventional care, but was only able to match 26 pairs of patients according to site of cancer and sex. In terms of quality of life, relatives claimed that hospice patients were more likely to have their pain relieved than hospital patients.

A similar approach was taken by Parkes and Parkes in their classic early evaluation of St Christopher's hospice (Parkes 1978, 1979, 1980, Parkes and Parkes 1984). In these studies patients were matched with others not receiving hospice care in terms of age, sex, socio-economic status, duration of terminal period, and severity of pain before the terminal period. In his study of an advisory domiciliary service Parkes (1980) was unable to detect any differences in perceived symptom control or quality of life between patients receiving or not receiving the home care service. Patients predominantly cared for at home (conventional care with no specialist palliative care input) experienced more pain than those dying in conventional hospitals, although there were important deficiencies in care in both settings (Parkes 1978). In a parallel study to evaluate the in-patient service, patients dying in the hospice had better pain control, were less likely to be confined to bed, and suffered less distress than patients receiving conventional hospital care (Parkes 1979). By the time this study was replicated 10 years later there was no longer any significant difference between the hospice and other hospitals, because the latter had improved considerably (Parkes and Parkes 1984).

The above studies using matched pairs provide very weak evidence. The effort made by Parkes to match patients on a number of variables led to small numbers of eligible patients, giving studies with little statistical power. This makes it likely that any significant differences in outcome between the models of care would not be detected. However complex the matching procedure, many other patient characteristics can act as potential confounding variables, and it is likely that different type of patients gained access to different types of healthcare. Finally, Parkes' studies were entirely based on retrospective interviews with surviving spouses, on average over a year after the patients' death. The problems previously discussed of the unreliability of relatives' assessments, the effects of the long delay on relatives' attitudes and recall, and the loyalty that relatives may have felt towards the hospice (as many remained involved with it) all raise doubts about the usefulness of these studies.

Addington-Hall *et al.* (1992) conducted a randomized controlled trial of nurses who were employed to co-ordinate the care of terminally ill cancer patients. One aim was to improve patients' quality of life through better co-ordination between the NHS, local authority services, and voluntary organizations. Although well conducted, this study illustrated many of the problems of palliative care research, with small numbers of patients, and high drop-out rates. The authors were unable to demonstrate important benefits in the care received by patients, possibly because the eventual power of the study was weak.

The most recent study to be reported is an evaluation by Higginson and Hearn (1997) of 11 multidisciplinary palliative care teams working in England or Ireland. The results suggest that the control of patients' pain improves after the involvement of the team, but this study has limitations because of the 'before and after' design and particularly the fact that the pain assessments were made by the team members providing the care.

Conclusions

In-patient and multisite services

There is evidence that in-patient palliative care results in better pain control compared with home care or conventional hospital care (Parkes 1978, 1979, Greer *et al.* 1986, Morris *et al.* 1986a, Seale 1991b). This conclusion is, however, based on research which is methodologically weak, and has not been supported in all studies (Kane *et al.* 1984). Several of the studies quoted are more than a decade old. In a follow-up to earlier studies, Parkes and Parkes (1984) showed that pain control had improved in both hospices and general hospitals, with a greater improvement in the latter, reducing previous differences.

Hospital palliative care support teams

There is limited evidence from non-experimental research that support teams can improve pain control (but no evidence about other quality of life measures) for patients dying in hospital (Ellershaw *et al.* 1995, McQuillan *et al.* 1996)

Home care

Until recently the limited research that had been conducted had not demonstrated that palliative home care teams, co-ordinating nurses, or advisory teams have an impact on the quality of life of patients dying at home (Parkes 1980, Zimmer *et al.* 1984, Zimmer *et al.* 1985, Addington-Hall *et al.* 1992, Dessloch *et al.* 1992, Hughes *et al.* 1992). An exception to this conclusion comes from the work of Wallston *et al.* (1988), who suggested that patients dying in home care hospices had better 'quality of death' than patients dying in hospital.

Ventafridda *et al.* (1989) suggested that patients cared for at home had better functional status than those treated in hospital. This finding in a small study may well be attributable to selection bias. The recent study by Higginson and Hearne (1997) provides the first evidence that community-based palliative care is beneficial in terms of pain control. This study is pragmatic, reflecting the reality of palliative care in several centres, and therefore has good general-izability. However, the strength of the evidence is limited for the reasons previously discussed.

There are several possible interpretations for these disappointing findings. It may be that these models of care do not in fact benefit patients in terms of quality of life. However, the limited nature of the research which has been conducted probably reflects the difficulties of carrying out research in this area. Most studies have been too small and methodologically weak to detect any differences which may exist. It is also possible that some previous evaluations have used inappropriate outcome measures which are too insensitive to detect the benefits achieved by palliative care.

Researchers must however resist the temptation to blame the lack of positive results on the evaluation tools used, but must devise and use tools which do reflect the aims of palliative care. There is a tendency in some of the literature to rationalize the negative results as unimportant, and to claim that the areas where positive results are found (e.g. a sense of involvement with care) are really the key aims of palliative medicine.

The aims of palliative medicine have been clearly defined (SMAC 1992, Johnston and Abraham 1995, Wiles 1995), and tools have been developed to assess the extent to which aims related to quality of life are met (Bruera *et al.* 1991, Higginson *et al.* 1992b, Higginson and McCarthy 1993, 1994, McMillan and Mahon 1994b, Cohen *et al.* 1997), thus addressing the claim that earlier quality of life scales may be inappropriate. It is not clear, however, that any of these assessment tools have achiever wide acceptance, mainly because of the length of time needed to complete them. Although the methodological difficulties must not be underestimated, there remains a need for research to evaluate all models of palliative care in terms of their impact on quality of life, if expansion of these forms of care is to be justified by evidence of effectiveness.

Question 8

Wider implications

ANNE NAYSMITH

What are the implications of alternative forms of service delivery for different sectors of the palliative care network, and for the wider use of resources?

Palliative care as a specialist discipline is relatively new. Not only has it developed in very different ways in different countries, and even in different parts of the same country, but it is also, as one would expect of a new discipline, undergoing continuous evolution. Studies of alternative forms of service delivery have therefore been difficult to conduct. It has rarely been considered ethical to randomize patients who wished to receive specialist palliative care if it meant depriving some of the trial group of that care. 'Before and after' studies have tended to involve small areas and low numbers of patients, so that there was considerable random variation in the baseline data, and to have been conducted against the background of a discipline in evolution so that changes were likely to be occurring which were not causally related to the variable under study. All this has made what data is available difficult to interpret with certainty.

Use of specialist palliative care services

In the UK, the majority of the research into the care of dying patients focuses on the work of specialist teams. However, it is important to recognize that the majority of home nursing services for the terminally ill are provided by district nurses (Seale 1992), and patients at home remain medically under the care of their general practitioner. Similarly, patients in hospital remain under the care of doctors in disciplines other than palliative medicine, and receive their nursing care from ward nurses (Hockley 1990).

Seale (1992) provided useful data on the home nursing provided to a random sample of 800 adults, chosen from 10 areas of England, who died in October and November 1987. Because this study replicated the methodology of an earlier study carried out in 1969 it was possible to make comparisons between the two time periods. In 1987, 12% of respondents felt they had needed nursing help at home but had not been offered it. Where nursing help was received, 22% of respondents would have preferred it to have been given more often (although only a quarter had requested this). In only 12% of cases did the district nurse feel that she would have liked to have visited more often. Where the answers of the respondent (usually the patient's main informal carer) and the district nurse could be directly compared, the respondent felt that more nursing help had been needed but this need was not recognized by the district nurse. These figures were surprisingly similar to the answers to these questions given in 1969, surprisingly because the pattern of nursing care at home had changed. In the 1987 study, people received less frequent visiting than in 1969, although the care was spread over a longer period of time. Educating informal carers to care for the patient at home appeared to have become a more important part of district nurses' work, allowing them to reduce their direct input. However, referrals were being made earlier before death.

It is often stated that the majority of people in the UK would prefer to die at home (National Council for Hospice and Specialist Palliative Care Services 1994), although in fact fewer and fewer people actually achieve this (Johnson and Oliver 1991). Were the trend towards institutional death to be reversed, the demand on general practitioners and district nursing services would need to be quantified, costed, and resourced.

The majority of patients in the UK who receive input from specialist palliative care services have cancer. Johnson and Oliver (1991) identified the proportion of cancer patients receiving care from a specialist service in one UK area in 1986–87. The community team, whose role was advisory, was involved in the care of 34% of all cancer deaths in Medway, but in 70% of the cases where death was at home. Additional patients received only in-patient hospice care, bringing the total specialist involvement to 43% of all cancer deaths. It is uncertain how far this figure could be increased by if specialist services were better resourced, as a substantial minority of cancer patients are not discharged from hospital between the diagnosis of advanced cancer and their death. A shift in the place of care away from acute hospitals would require a corresponding and significant move of resources.

Specialist palliative care support teams to help patients in the community have been established in many areas. There are wide differences in the way in which these support teams work, in part reflecting their management structure and source of funding. Lunt and Yardley (1988) carried out a major study of 50 home care teams in the UK, in which he documented their work load in 1985–86. The case-load per nurse specialist varied from 11–57 with a mean of 21. The stated aim of the teams was to act as a resource for primary healthcare teams and hospital staff.

Hospital-based support teams have similar aims (Hockley 1990). However, most of the nurse specialists felt they were most effective when working directly with patients. Differences between paediatric oncology nurse specialists were even more marked (Hunt 1995). Nurses based in district paediatric services carried out substantial amounts of direct patient care for children with a variety of diseases. However, nurses based at regional paediatric centres, many of whom were funded by Macmillan Cancer Relief, spent a high proportion of their time in educational activity and acting as a secondary resource, and tended to care wholly or substantially for cancer patients. Sadly, studies are lacking into the comparative cost-effectiveness of alternative models.

Only a small minority of patients who die from diseases other than cancer receive care from specialist palliative care services, although these patients are often similarly symptomatic. There are widespread fears that encouraging the referral of patients with non-malignant diseases to specialist services would increase demand to a level which could not possibly be met within existing resources, but data on the needs of these patients and their carers is scanty. One study using 14 general practices in Derbyshire (Kurti and O'Dowd 1995) identified 20 carers of patients who had died of a non-malignant terminal illness. The patients had been cared for at home for an average of 5.3 years (range 5 months to 15 years). Not surprisingly, tiredness was the major problem identified by carers. In this very small sample, the length of time patients were cared for was longer than for patients with cancer, and it seemed difficult for the primary healthcare team to identify the point at which their care became palliative. Were this sample to be representative of patients dying of non-malignant diseases, it would imply that it might be more difficult for specialist services to identify the point at which their involvement could be appropriate, and the greater duration of the terminal illness would imply a higher cost per patient.

Development of specialist palliative care services

UK

Ignoring detailed local differences, specialist palliative care services may be taken to comprise community support teams, day care, hospital support teams, and specialist in-patient units (National Council for Hospice and Specialist Palliative Care Services 1994). It is rare for all these components to be within a single unit of management, and even more rare for all the components to be developed at the same time. It would be tempting to suppose that the development of a specialist service could substitute days in home or hospice care for days in acute hospital care and death at home for death in an institution, and that this would lead to cost savings.

There are few British studies. Johnson and Oliver (1991) studied the site of death of all cancer patients dying in Medway between 1977 and 1988. The introduction of a community support team in 1978 led to a transient increase in the number of deaths at home (and therefore fewer in hospital). When a specialist palliative care in-patient unit was opened in 1984 there was a sharp rise in the number of deaths in the unit but only a slight further fall in the number of hospital deaths. The major change was a substitution of hospice deaths (at higher cost) for home deaths, although in later years there was a slight recovery in the proportion of home deaths.

Although a terminal admission may be precipitated by an acute clinical problem, it is often because the informal carers can no longer carry the physical and emotional burden of the patient's care. The provision of continuous home nursing might relieve this burden and avoid admission. The introduction of a new home nursing service in Bristol (Robbins *et al.* 1997) allowed 62 of the 64 patients who received the service to die at home. However, there was no discernible change in the overall number of patients known to the home support team who died at home. This may have been because the new service was too small to produce a measurable impact, but it may also have been because it produced a higher quality of care for a group of families already highly motivated to achieve a home death, rather than substituting for in-patient care. The service was highly rated both by informal carers and by the primary healthcare team. But if these patients were likely to die at home under any circumstances the costs of the new service, which were comparable to in-patient care, were an addition to the overall costs of palliative care rather than a substitution of one type of care for another. A similar service for patients with HIV disease in inner London did significantly increase the proportion of patients dying at home, but from a very low starting point and in a highly selected group, many of whom had no informal carer (Koffman *et al.* 1996).

Bennett and Corcoran (1994) documented the effect of introducing a hospital support team on the workload of the community support team in the surrounding area. Few patients were referred to the hospital team more than 3 months before death. Nevertheless, during the first 4 years from the establishment of the hospital support team there was a progressive increase both in the number of patients referred to the community support team and in the interval between referral and death. There was no change in these parameters for patients referred by their general practitioner. The increased workload was entirely due to referrals from the hospital support team. Over this period there was no significant increase in the interval between referral to the hospital support team and death. In many cases the patient was referred as soon as recurrent or metastatic cancer was diagnosed, so that the interval between referral and death was also the interval between diagnosis and death. This interval could not therefore be lengthened.

North America

Hospice programmes have developed rather differently in the USA. Predominantly home-based, they offer intensive home visiting, home nursing, and in some cases specialist in-patient care from a single unified service which tends to be seen as a substitute for conventional care rather than as an addition. Patients enrolled in hospice programmes tend to have fewer aggressive treatment interventions (Wachtel and Mor 1987), to spend fewer days in an acute hospital (Brooks and SmythStaruch 1984, McCusker and Stoddard 1987), and, if in a home-based hospice programme without attached in-patient beds, tend to die at home (Kidder 1992). There is a measurable substitution of home visiting for hospital in-patient care (Brooks and SmythStaruch 1984, McCusker and Stoddard 1987).

Hospice care is self-selected. In comparative research studies the hospice patient population is therefore unlikely to be fully comparable with control groups who did not receive hospice care. Data suggests hospice patients are likely to have been diagnosed longer and to have a greater level of informal support. Other possible factors, such as the patient's attitude to aggressive therapeutic interventions prior to diagnosis, are almost impossible to assess (Kidder 1992).

Australia

The home support team service of Western Sydney was extended by the provision of an out-of-hours on-call nursing service. It was hoped that this would reduce acute hospital admissions. However, there was no significant change either in the number of hospital admissions or in the length of stay. There was a trend towards admitting patients to local hospitals rather than the tertiary cancer centre after the introduction of the programme. During this study the on-call nurses were not allowed to administer drugs additional to the patients' existing therapy, which limited their ability to intervene. No significant cost savings were demonstrated (Aristides and Shiell 1993).

Overall effects on total workload

The implication of these studies is that there is no simple substitution of specialist palliative care for conventional care. Rather, as additional components of a complete specialist palliative care service (Neale *et al.* 1993) are put in place in a defined area the total workload of all components taken together tends to increase, and a number of patients will receive care from more than one component of the service during the course of their illness. In the UK, the period in which the provision of in-patient hospice beds has expanded rapidly has also been the period when the number of acute hospital beds has decreased markedly in many areas. Although hospice care is often less costly per bed night than acute hospital care, in the context of a shrinking hospital sector it is not possible to identify the provision of in-patient hospice care as a substitution for conventional care. There are suggestions from both British (Hockley 1992) and American (Kidder 1992) studies that, when specialist palliative in-patient beds are provided, the proportion of patients dying at home falls.

Costs of palliative care

None of the papers reviewed allowed us to calculate the costs of palliative care in general. There are few data on the costs of specialist palliative care in the UK. Because of the funding structure of the NHS, there are no patient-based sources of routine data identifying the costs of a complete illness. Research attempting to quantify these costs for a sample of patients is difficult to carry out, because patients move between care settings and become increasingly unable to provide information as they enter the most expensive part of their illness, the period leading up to death.

Such data as is available in the UK identifies the additional costs generated by a specific specialist palliative care service. Lovel (1996) costed a specialist medical assessment visit at £125 in the patient's home and £75 in hospital in 1996. Only 30% of patients assessed required admission to a specialist in-patient unit; the remainder had their symptoms controlled as a result of the advice given. However, there was no data on cost-effectiveness.

The provision of extended nursing care in Bristol (Robbins *et al.* 1997) cost £80 000 in direct costs for 77 patient episodes in the first year, an average of £389.31 per patient or £8.11 per nursing hour. Indirect costs, which were absorbed by the parent institutions, were not quantified. Since each episode of care averaged little more than 48 hours, and in-patient care was costed at £160 upwards per day, there would have been no savings even had care at home substituted for in-patient care. Since admission rates did not alter significantly, these were again additional costs.

Introducing the on-call nursing service in Western Sydney (Aristides and Shiell 1993) cost A$580 000 per annum. This investment produced at best a saving of A$700 per patient for the 123 patients covered by the service. Cost-effectiveness was again not demonstrated, the costs of the service being essentially added to conventional care.

Much better data on the costs of hospice care are available from the US. Not all cost changes are savings. Goldberg *et al.* (1986) reported data on drug use from the National Hospice Study. Only 57% of terminally ill patients in conventional care were taking opioids for analgesia. This rose to 85% of home hospice and 90% of in-patient hospice patients. Similar trends are likely for other drugs such as anti-emetics. Although counterbalanced by the reduced number of aggressive therapeutic interventions (40% of hospice patients vs 50% of conventional care patients), these findings suggest that drug costs may be higher in patients receiving specialist palliative care. No direct measurements were made of the effectiveness or cost-effectiveness of the prescribed analgesia.

A number of studies have attempted to measure the total costs of care during terminal cancer for both hospice and conventional care patients in the US, aided by the availability of Medicare and insurance information on reimbursements. Although hospice patients spent fewer days in hospital, these savings were counterbalanced by the much higher level of home visits to hospice patients. Savings only became apparent if hospital admission could be avoided in the last weeks of life (Brooks and SmythStaruch 1984), and were negated if patients remained for long periods in hospice programmes, e.g. more than 5 months (McCusker and Stoddard 1987). High intensity home care was as expensive as conventional hospital care (McCusker and Stoddard 1987). For patients in whom hospital admission was prevented by home hospice care (Brooks and Smyth-Staruch 1984), hospice costs of $203 per patient for the last 2 weeks of life saved $1270 of conventional health costs; similarly, hospice costs of $862 per patient for the last 12 weeks of life saved on average $3480 per patient.

Patients with HIV disease pose a particular problem because of the high costs of their care. Many American hospice programmes have difficulty caring for substantial numbers because of the cost (Tehan 1991) and are exploring methods of inter-agency working in order to share the expenditure across as wide a range of funding sources as possible (Shapiro 1988). Other non-malignant diseases in the terminal phase may also turn out to have very different costs.

The costs of palliative care cannot necessarily be extrapolated from the experience with cancer patients.

Substantial savings might be made if high-technology care for dying patients could be avoided, since in the majority of patients it is futile. Advance directives were thought to offer a way in which patients could decline inappropriate care in advance (Singer and Lowy 1992). However, the patients who make advance directives may well be disinclined in any case to accept hospitalization or aggressive interventions (Weeks *et al.* 1994), and estimates of the true savings to be made in the US are of the order of 25% of the costs of terminal hospital admissions (Weeks *et al.* 1994). In the UK aggressive interventions are less often offered to the terminally ill, so that much smaller savings are likely to be available. Similarly, a study of patients with advanced cancer admitted to intensive care in the US showed that 79% either died in hospital or spent less than 3 months at home before death (Schapira *et al.* 1993). No good prognostic factors were identified to select those likely to benefit from intensive care. Overall, it has been estimated that encouraging advance directives, avoiding therapy which can be predicted to be futile, and developing home hospice programmes could at best save 3.3% of US health costs (Emanuel and Emanuel 1994).

These savings do not take into account the costs to patients, families, and informal carers, on whom the main burden of care falls during home hospice care. Studies of the costs of hospice care in the US confirm that the main costs are borne by the informal carers of patients in home hospice care, who give 10–16 hours of care a day. These costs vary widely. Many patients and their carers have retired before cancer develops; they do not lose income, and the main cost is the notional wage earned by the informal carers. If the main carer has to give up work or become a part-time worker, financial losses are substantial, including not only loss of salary but also of pension rights, savings etc., and the possibility of becoming dependent on benefits. The average financial costs to families are at least equal to the cost of caring for the patient in a nursing home (Muurinen 1986, Stommel *et al.* 1993). In the UK, where few palliative care services can offer as much care at home as typical American programmes, it is likely that costs to families are of a similar or higher order. As demographic change begins to produce fewer informal carers able to take on this burden of unpaid care, the challenge to health and social expenditure is likely to increase.

Conclusion

Palliative care support teams have as their stated aim to act as a secondary resource for community and hospital staff. In the UK they are involved with around half of all dying cancer patients, but very small numbers of patients with non-malignant disease. The limited evidence available suggests that most provide a service which is additional to conventional care, which is greatly appreciated by patients and families but whose cost-effectiveness has not been demonstrated.

Patients often receive care from several components of a specialist palliative care service. Developing any one part of a palliative care service is likely to increase workload for all parts.

Where in-patient palliative care beds are provided, the number of patients dying at home tends to decrease. It is increasingly difficult to prevent patients from being admitted to hospital or hospice for terminal care. Intensive home care services have not been shown in general to increase the proportion of patients dying at home and may be as expensive as in-patient care.

Informal carers provide most of the care for dying patients and are essential if substantial numbers of people are to die at home. No account is taken of the cost of this to patients and families. It is important to note that future demographic change may reduce the availability of informal carers, which will have implications for the provision of palliative care.

Question 9

Palliative care in hospital

SUZANNE KITE

How can different models of organization or bed utilization improve the care of patients dying in hospital?

This chapter is based on a review of 62 papers relating to the care of people dying in hospital. There were very few papers evaluating different models of palliative care provision within hospitals, and the more informative of these are summarized in Table 9.1. A significant number of papers documented existing deficiencies in the care of patients dying in hospital, with recommendations for improvement. The development of different services in response to local need are well described.

The majority of papers were published in the UK or the US. Cost-effectiveness of the different models of care receives little detailed attention, and is confined to the American studies. A review of the background literature is presented here, before moving on to consider the few evaluative studies in depth.

Establishing the need for hospital-based palliative care services

The proportion of people who die in hospital is steadily rising. Approximately two-thirds of all deaths now occur in institutions, predominantly in acute hospitals (Cartwright 1991a). Only 10% of people die unexpectedly (Lunt 1980, McGuire *et al.* 1994), and the majority of deaths occur after a prolonged period of illness, with acute hospitals also playing a greater role towards the end of life (Cartwright 1991a). Wherever they may die, people are increasingly likely to be admitted to hospital during the last year of their life, whether it be for a number of short stays, continuing care when living at home is no longer possible, or a period of terminal care (Cartwright 1991a, Tarr *et al.* 1992, Wilkes 1984). The causes of

Table 9.1   Informative and evaluative studies of hospital care services

Author	Countries	Intervention and year (s) of data collection	Study design and research setting	Subjects	Outcome measures
McQuillan *et al.* (1996)	UK	Symptom control in a teaching hospital before and after introduction of a palliative care registrar 1991–93	Before and after questionnaire study Teaching hospital	In-patients with diagnosis of cancer or HIV/AIDS Total no. 366 193 cancer 173 HIV/ AIDS	Pain control Professional's opinion Prescribing levels Symptom control
Ellershaw *et al.* (1995)	UK	Prospective study of cancer patients referred to King's College Hospital 1992	Observational study Teaching hospital	Patients with malignant disease (cancer) referred to PCT Total no. 125 68 male 57 female median age 68 years (range 14–90) 1 group only	Patients' placements Patient and relative insight Symptom control

Measurement tools	Results	Key conclusions	Comments
Symptom control questionnaire for patients Questionnaire for health professionals.- views on protocols and palliative care registrar	Statistically significant changes in analgesic prescribing, with increased use of subcutaneous diamorphine ($p < 0.008$), NSAIDS ($p = 0.02$), and reduced use of inappropriate opioids, other than pethidine ($p = 0.004$) Patients' problems on admission were similar during both surveys but, after introduction of PCT fewer patients reported a deterioration in their pain scores (not statistically significant) Trends to improvement for nausea, vomiting, constipation and sore mouth. 53% response rate to hospital staff questionnaire: 90% of respondents found the palliative medicine registrar helpful	Staff value the service. Cohort one third size necessary to demon-strate statistically significant changes of order expected in symptom control and prescribing habits.staff found educational guidelines helpful, but used them infrequently	Strengths: Studied patient symptom reports; groups before and after intervention comparable; excellent patient response rate (88% overall) Weaknesses: Lack of statistical power. Poor hospital staff response rate (53%)
PACA palliative care assessment tool	Within 4 days of PCT involvement there were statistically significant improvements in pain control ($p < 0.001$), nausea ($p < 0.009$), insomnia ($p < 0.004$), and anorexia ($p < 0.001$), maintained at day 7 at which time relief of constipation was also achieved ($p < 0.02$) Also significant change in insight of patients ($p < 0.001$) and relatives ($p < 0.02$) Appropriate placement assisted by interventions undertaken by the team	Hospital PCT is effective at improving symptom control, facilitates understand-ing of the diagnosis and prognosis, and con-tributes to the appropriate placement of patients	Strengths: Studied patients' symptom reports. Validity and reliability of PACA tool demonstrated Weaknesses: Structure and working pattern of PCT not clearly described. Number of patients unable to complete questionnaires during study period not stated

Table 9.1   (contd)

Author	Countries	Intervention and year (s) of data collection	Study design and research setting	Subjects	Outcome measures
Kane *et al.* (1984)	USA	Hospice care compared to conventional care at a veterans' hospital Year of data collection not known	Randomized control trial Veterans' hospital	Largely male veterans, all with cancer Total no. 247 Mean age 64 (range 34–92) 137 hospice 110 control	Bed utilization Carer satisfaction Costs Functional status Length of stay Life expectancy Satisfaction Prescribing Psychological status Quality of life Pain/ symptom control
Bruera (1989)	Canada	Before and after the establishment of a pain and symptom control team 1984 and 1987	Before and after study Cancer care unit	All cancer patients Total no. 200 100 in 1984 group, mean age 55 yrs (±17) 100 in 1987 group, mean age 58 yrs (±14)	Length of stay Non-pharmaco-logic treatment of pain Pain control Prescribing levels

PCT, palliative care team; PSCT, pain and symptom control team

Measurement tools	Results	Key conclusions	Comments
Activity of Daily Living Index; Adapted symptom scale Pain Assessment Profile; Anxiety scale: Rand Health Insurance Study CES-D Depression Scale; McCaffree & Harkins Physical- Environment Scale; McGill Pain Questionnaire; National Cancer Institutes Hospice Study involvement- in-care questions; Quality of life index; Ware Satisfaction Scale.	No significant differences between hospice and conventional care in terms of: survival curves; total no. of in-patient days; proportion receiving anti- cancer treatment; pain and symptom control; anxiety and depression. Hospice patients were significant more satisfied with interpersonal care ($p < 0.01$) and involvement in care ($p < 0.01$) Family members of hospice patients showed less anxiety and more satisfaction with involvement in care There were no significant differences in overall costs for hospice and control groups	Hospice care provides an appropriate alternative form of therapy for terminally ill people, but is compara- tively no better or worse than conven-tional care	Strengths: Relatively complete follow up achieved. Sample size based on pre-study considerations of statistical power Weaknesses: Method of randomization not stated. Validity of adapted question- naires not stated. Patients and fami- lies not representa- tive of the general population. Too many confounding variables in the degree of hospice care received by the two groups
Data from medical and nursing records	Average daily dose parenteral morphine per patient was higher in 1987 than 1984 ($p < 0.05$) Parenteral narcotics were prescribed subcutaneously in 0/52 cases in 1984 versus 21/ 63 cases in 1987 (33%, $p < 0.01$) The pattern of prescription of narcotics by residents changed significantly during the last 4 weeks of rotation compared to the first few weeks No significant change in prescription of antiemetics, laxatives and regular versus intermittent prescription of analgesics	Some changes in modality of treatment of pain may be attributable to PSCT via education of residents, and continued improvement in assessment of pain by nurses. However in several areas of treatment the impact of the PSCT remains minimal	Strengths: Samples in 1984 and 1987 appropriate and comparable, recruited consecutively. Statistical methods described and appropriate. Overall conclusions justified Weaknesses; Retrospective study, using nurse records to assess pain

these trends are multifactorial, but the increasing number of deaths in the elderly (Cartwright 1991a), and the continuous development of medical technology, are likely to be major factors.

The palliative care needs of those dying in hospital were first addressed in the literature in the 1970s and early 1980s, with the recognition that the bulk of the work of caring for the terminally ill was done by ordinary general hospitals and community services, rather than by specialist hospice teams (Hinton 1979, Lunt 1980, Lunt and Hillier 1981, Wilkes 1984). The need to disseminate hospice skills to all dying patients was stressed. A subsequent DHSS Circular (Anonymous 1984a), and a report from the National Association of Health Authorities (Boomla 1987), both called for an examination of the services provided for dying patients and their relatives in hospital.

Research clearly demonstrated the need for strategies to improve the care of patients dying in hospital. Poor pain and symptom control was documented repeatedly in 50–70% of patients dying in hospital, prior to the establishment of palliative care services (Hockley *et al.* 1988, Simpson 1991, Tarr *et al.* 1992). The inappropriate use of medication for symptom control was also well described (Addington Hall *et al.* 1991, Hockley *et al.* 1988, Higginson *et al.* 1990, Simpson 1991, Mills *et al.* 1994). Most patients were found to have multiple symptoms (Simpson 1991). Qualitative research reinforced these findings (Mills *et al.* 1994).

Studies investigating the wider provision of palliative care provided insight into the satisfaction of patients and carers with hospital services. Higginson *et al.* (1990) interviewed 65 terminally ill cancer patients and their families in the community. A quarter of patients and carers were dissatisfied with communication with hospital doctors and nurses, and 17% of patients and 11% of family members felt that hospital services were poorly co-ordinated. Hospital staff were perceived to be overworked. A specific recommendation was made for improved undergraduate training in the breaking of bad news.

Comments on hospital doctors and nurses

Positive comments were general ('smashing', 'caring', 'kind') or specific ('I liked the doctor who broke bad news by holding my hand and stroking it'). Negative comments related to three main issues. Communication with doctors and nurses was the subject most commonly mentioned and was usually related to previous rather than current difficulties—for example, 'The ward sister told me abruptly, in front of my wife, that I had 2 months to live'; 'The consultant sat on the end of the bed, swung his legs and said "Well, you've got cancer".' Patients and family members found it difficult to ask questions—for example, 'Hospital doctors stand there with information in their head and expect you to read their mind. Very high and mighty, one or two of them.' Some patients and family members understood that their doctors had difficulty dealing with aspects of death and dying: 'The doctors were good but too glib. To surgeons, as I'm dying I'm a failure. I often embarrass them.' Greater honesty would have been preferred: 'They were a bit optimistic over the nerve block; they said very confidently it would work ... it would have been better to be more honest.' Two patients said they had not been told what was wrong with them in hospital.

Co-ordination of services was commented on by 11 patients and seven family members. Their complaints included past delays in the outpatient department of waiting for ambulances and ill informed doctors and nurses.

Overworked staff was the third issue eliciting negative comment. Doctors and nurses were described by five subjects as 'too busy to have time to care'. One family member suggested that 'there should be more nursing assistants to deal with the bed making, etc, and registered nurses might do better to circulate more slowly rather than bustling between one demanding patient and the next, and overlooking the quiet patients.' (Higginson *et al.* 1990)

In a retrospective interview survey of carers of patients with cancer dying in hospital, Addington-Hall *et al.* (1991) found that half of the carers had complaints about the hospital care received, with a third of this group stating that nurses were too busy to provide adequate care. Inadequate information provided by the hospital was another common problem (39%), and, specifically, 10% had wanted to know more about the timing of death. The National Hospice study, conducted in the US and based on the recollections of carers, suggested that the care of those dying in hospital might be improved in a number of ways. These included earlier recognition of terminal patients, with greater consideration of the appropriateness of diagnostic tests and aggressive treatments in this group; greater access to social service support and liaison with community services, to reduce financial hardship and increase the possibility of dying at home, and improved symptom control (Greer *et al.* 1986, Wallston *et al.* 1988). The limitations of retrospective studies, using proxies as informants, apply to both of these last studies.

Different models of care

The various models of palliative care provision developed within hospitals have already been described in Question 3. The discussion here will focus on studies which have attempted to evaluate these different services.

The only published randomized controlled trial of hospital-based palliative care services involved a comparison between a composite mix of services against conventional care (Kane *et al.* 1984, 1985a). The authors evaluated hospice care for cancer patients at the Veterans Administration Hospital, University of California, Los Angeles (UCLA). Hospice care in this context referred to a palliative care programme comprising an 11 bedded in-patient unit, home-care, and an hospital-wide consultation service for patients under the care of other teams. The 247 patients in the study group were predominantly elderly male veterans. Patients were recruited if the admitting physician estimated their prognosis to be between 2 weeks and 6 months, and if the patient was aware of their prognosis and consented to inclusion. Patients were then randomly assigned to receive hospice or conventional care. During the study no subjects were admitted to the hospice programme except through the process of informed consent and randomization. Baseline and follow-up interviews and multidimensional questionnaires were used for assessment with patients and familial care-givers, according to a fixed schedule until death or until an upper limit of interviews had been completed, (see Table 9.1).

The results of the UCLA study caused considerable impact and debate, as they reported no significant differences between hospice and conventional care in terms of pain and symptom control; anxiety and depression; total number of in-patient days; survival curves, or the proportion of patients receiving anti-cancer treatment. They did, however, find that hospice patients were significantly more satisfied with interpersonal care and involvement with care, and that family members of hospice patients showed less anxiety and more satisfaction with involvement in care. There were no significant differences in overall costs for hospice and control groups. Kane concluded that although hospice care did provide an appropriate alternative form of therapy for terminally ill people, it was comparatively no better or worse than conventional care (Kane *et al.* 1984).

However, these results need to be interpreted with caution in the light of observations on the study methods as well as on more general issues (Mahoney 1986, Seale 1989). The validity of the outcome measures has been questioned (Mahoney 1986, Seale 1989), and any steps taken to validate the adapted tools in this population are not stated. In the absence of baseline information on the different services offered at UCLA, the similarity in the proportions of patients receiving specific anti-cancer treatment, diagnostic investigations and survival curves could be due to considerable overlap between the two groups, that is they may be drawn from the same population. If so, these are inappropriate outcome measures, and lend support to the concerns about the separation of treatment and control arms. Hospice patients received care in the same hospital as the control patients and some 'hospice' patients received care from both hospital and hospice physicians. Hospice physicians gave advice, but did not prescribe, to patients outside the in-patient unit. According to Mahoney (1986), 37 of the 137 'hospice' patients were never under the direct care of the hospice physician, and only 24 of the hospice patients were under direct hospice care for more than 75% of the time. No information is given on where the hospice patients received their diagnostic tests and anti-cancer treatment, and whether the intention was curative or palliative. By assessing the entire hospice programme collectively, and with little background information, particularly on home care, it is impossible to assess the impact of the component parts or to interpret the results meaningfully. Neither is it clear how long the hospice program had been running, and the degree to which it had been assimilated into the hospital—with potential benefits to the other hospital patients. Education and skill-sharing are intrinsic to palliative care, and one would expect the experience gained in specialist palliative care units to be disseminated locally, as shown by Murray Parkes (Parkes and Parkes 1984).

Mahoney (1986) makes two other useful observations on the UCLA study. Firstly, if nursing home days are included, then the hospice patients spent 46% of their time at home, compared to 39% of those receiving conventional care. Secondly, he notes that quality of life scores were averaged for patients at different stages of illness and with variable proximity to death, which makes interpretation of these results difficult.

Finally, even the findings of the UCLA study and Kane's conclusions are accepted, it is difficult to generalize the results when the study population was so unrepresentative of the general population, or of the group of patients usually referred to palliative care teams.

Hospital support teams

The most common response to the evident need for improved care for those dying in hospital has been the development of multi-disciplinary palliative care teams. By 1997, 139 hospital palliative care teams had been established in the UK and Ireland (Hospice Information Service 1997a). Such teams may variably be described as 'support teams', 'palliative care teams', or 'symptom control teams' in the UK, or under the umbrella term 'hospice' within the United States, but they share the basic model described in Question 3.

The potential advantages of this model of a hospital support team are well described. By working alongside other hospital staff, there are opportunities to share and disseminate palliative care skills widely, without de-skilling those working in other specialities. Patients can benefit from a palliative care approach at an earlier stage of illness than that conventionally seen in hospices or by community teams. Guidelines on certain aspects of symptom control can be formulated in response to local need (Hockley 1996, McQuillan *et al.* 1996). Although costings are rarely cited in the literature, such a model is relatively inexpensive, and there is the potential for saving money by reducing in-patient stay through improved pain and symptom control, and the facilitation of discharge planning (Bates *et al.* 1981, O'Neill *et al.* 1992).

The main disadvantages of hospital support teams are the potential confusion over responsibility for patient care, and the demanding nature of shared care, well demonstrated in the account of the short life of the terminal care support team at Charing Cross Hospital, London (Herxheimer *et al.* 1985).

Whereas the establishment and early development of hospital support teams have been covered well in the literature, there is less documented evidence of their effectiveness. Hockley *et al.* (1988) and Lickiss *et al.* (1994) both cite indirect evidence of effectiveness in the steady pattern of increased referrals to their respective teams. Hockley *et al.* (1988) note that 1 year after the introduction of the team, the number of complaints made by relatives about the care of the dying in the hospital had fallen from 14 to 5 per annum. Lickiss *et al.* (1994) also comment on the improved use of opiates within the hospital since the inception of the team.

More formal evaluations of hospital support teams have only been published recently, possibly because energy was initially focused on establishing the need, and then on developing the service. The evidence currently available is limited and consists of a prospective study (Ellershaw *et al.* 1995); one prospective and two retrospective before-and-after comparisons (Bruera 1989, Woodruff *et al.* 1991, McQuillan *et al.* 1996), and a small case–control study (Mortenson *et al.* 1983). The development of an audit tool is also described (Latimer 1991). The most informative of these studies are included in Table 9.1 and are discussed below.

Ellershaw *et al.* (1995) conducted a prospective study of 125 hospital in-patients with malignant disease, referred to King's College Hospital (London) advisory palliative care team. King's College Hospital is a teaching hospital with 600 acute beds. They designed a palliative care assessment tool (PACA) in order to assess the outcome of interventions made within 2 weeks of referral with regard to symptom control, change in the patients' and their relatives' insight regarding diagnosis and prognosis, and facilitation of patient placement. The validity and reliability of the PACA tool are demonstrated using appropriate methods. The study included all patients with malignant disease referred to the team from May to October 1992. Patients were assessed, by doctors and nurses on the team, at referral and then twice weekly over the subsequent 2 week period, unless the patient was discharged or died. The highly significant improvements in pain and symptom control, as well as changes in the insight of patients, and the successful involvement of the team in placement issues, led the authors to conclude that a hospital palliative care team can make a significant contribution to patient care. The direct questioning of patients, rather than using proxies, increases the validity of the results. However, the proportion of patients remaining in the study dropped to 70% at day 4, to 53% at day 7, and to 22% at day 13, and it is not clear whether this reflects losses due to deaths and discharges, or whether a number of patients were unwilling or unable to participate in the assessments. This information would be useful given the acknowledged difficulties of using formal assessment tools with terminally ill patients, and might substantiate or tend to refute the claim that the PACA form is concise and easy to complete. The lack of a control group means that we do not know whether such improvements in patient care would have been observed without the intervention of the team. However, it is difficult to define what a suitable control group would have been, as randomization of such an established service would have caused ethical and practical difficulties. There would have been similar difficulties in identifying controls for a case–control study. In any event, the evidence from work done by Simpson (1991) and others suggests that such marked improvements in symptom control are not observed without palliative care intervention. There is also the question of interviewer bias, but to employ external interviewers might have been intrusive to a vulnerable group of patients.

Overall, this study is important as the first, and only, formal evaluation of an established hospital palliative care team, providing evidence of the effectiveness of this model in this location. The PACA tool is also an important development in that it could be applied in other hospitals to evaluate team effectiveness, to obtain a rapid overview of each patient, and to facilitate communication within the team.

The study by McQuillan *et al.* (1996), coupled with the survey of the incidence of symptoms in cancer patients admitted to the University Hospital of Wales by Tarr *et al.* (1992), constitutes a before-and-after trial of the effects of the introduction of a palliative care service employing a doctor and part-time pharmacist. The doctor was available to see and advise about terminally ill patients, and collaborated with the pharmacist on an educational programme of meetings, teaching sessions, and information leaflets. This model deviates from the classical multidisciplinary team presented earlier. One year after the introduction of this service a repeat survey was conducted of all cancer and HIV in-patients. Patients were recruited over a 1 month period and followed for 6 weeks. Patients were interviewed and asked to rate symptoms, and those that were too ill to be interviewed were excluded. The initial interview was within 72 hours of admission, and was then repeated at weekly intervals throughout the patients' stay. Questionnaires were also issued to staff to assess their satisfaction with the service.

Patients' symptoms on admission were similar during both surveys but, after the introduction of the palliative care service, fewer patients reported a deterioration in their pain scores (not statistically significant), and there were trends towards improvement in nausea, vomiting, constipation, and sore mouth. The initial patient response rate to the interviews was excellent (88%). There were statistically significant changes in analgesic prescribing, particularly in the use of opiates. The majority of hospital staff responding to the questionnaire found the palliative medicine registrar helpful, and found the educational guidelines informative but used them infrequently. The authors draw attention to the cohort size, which was judged on pre-study considerations of statistical power to be one-third of the size necessary to demonstrate significant changes of the order expected in symptom control and prescribing habits, but the duration of the study was limited by financial considerations. Therefore, the effectiveness of the team in symptom control may be underestimated. Patients were interviewed by ward pharmacists, who were not palliative care team members, thus making interviewer bias a less likely explanation for the positive trends. The authors acknowledge that the effectiveness of a palliative care service is judged on more than symptom control, and limit their conclusions on the impact of the service to a probable improvement in prescribing and symptom control, and to being valued by staff. Whether palliative care doctors working outside the multidisciplinary structure in the hospital setting can adequately address the psychological, social, and dependency problems of patients is debatable (Meystre *et al.* 1996).

The two other before-and-after studies were conducted retrospectively, and used chart reviews rather than the views of patients themselves, both significant methodological weaknesses (Bruera 1989, Woodruff *et al.* 1991). Bruera in Edmonton, Canada, compared patients treated in a cancer centre in 1984 with the same number of patients treated in 1987, after the establishment of a pain and symptom control team (PSCT) (Bruera 1989). There were significant changes in the prescription of opiates, but there were no significant changes in the prescription of anti-emetics, laxatives and regular versus as-required analgesics. The pattern of prescribing of opioids by residents changed significantly during their attachment to the cancer centre. The authors conclude that the PSCT may have influenced the treatment of pain via the education of residents, and the continued improvement in the assessment of pain by nurses, but in several areas of treatment the impact of the PSCT remained minimal. They identify the need for the intensive teaching of pain and symptom management to residents as a key to improved patient care, as they usually manage pain control in large centres.

Woodruff *et al.* (1991) retrospectively reviewed the notes of the 241 patients referred to the palliative care service in a general teaching hospital in Australia during its first year of operation, and compared these with an earlier retrospective study at the hospital (Chan and Woodruff 1991). They cite improved pain control, and an increased number of patients enabled to die at home, as evidence of the success of the team, but reviewer bias and the differences between the two patient groups studied are not discussed.

One other study demonstrates the impact of a hospital palliative care team. Bennett and Corcoran (1994) studied the effect of such a team, based at a large teaching hospital in Leeds, England, on the surrounding community palliative care service They found that the establishment of the hospital team markedly increased the workload of the home care team, by both increasing the total number of referrals to the community service, and by referring patients earlier in their illness than did local general practitioners. This suggests that the hospital team is an effective model for improving access to specialist palliative care services.

Hospital support nurses

In addition to hospital support teams, there were 176 hospital support nurses working independently in the UK and Ireland in 1996 (Hospice Information Service 1997a). Such clinical nurse specialists may be employed to provide general palliative care, or supportive care within particular departments. These models of care have been poorly covered in the literature.

The results of the SUPPORT (Study to Understand Prognoses and Preferences for Outcomes and Risks of Treatments) trial, conducted in the US, highlight the challenges that such clinical nurse specialists may face (Connors *et al.* 1995). This randomized trial aimed to improve end-of-life decision-making and to reduce the frequency of a mechanically supported, painful, and prolonged process of dying, by improving communication between physicians and patients and families via a specialist nurse. However, the intervention of this specialist nurse did not lead to changes in established practice or improvements in the deficiencies of care for seriously ill, hospitalized patients. The authors conclude that greater individual commitment and societal education and debate are needed to improve care in these patients. In a subsequent commentary on the study, Curtin (1996) hypothesizes that the results may also reflect the limited voice that nurses may have within hierarchical, medical structures.

Hospice units in the hospital setting

There is a surprising dearth of published information about hospice units in acute hospital settings. There are comments on the development of such units (Hoskin and Hanks 1988, Severs and Wilkins 1991) but no evidence of evaluation. The same is true of the 'scattered beds' model of in-patient specialist palliative care. There is the suggestion that patients cared for in either of these settings are more likely to receive diagnostic procedures and specific tumor-icidal therapy than those in conventional hospice settings (Hannan and O'Donnell 1984, Greer *et al.* 1986, Hoskin and Hanks 1988). Depending on the specific situation and author, such treatment can be interpreted as necessary for effective symptom control (Hoskin and Hanks 1988) or unnecessarily burdensome (Greer *et al.* 1986), and expensive (Patton and Mooney 1990). Qualitative research suggests that integration of hospice units within hospitals can lead to a dilution of hospice philosophy, with a shift in emphasis from psychosocial to physical care (Seale 1989).

Day hospital

The role of day hospitals in the care of patients receiving palliative care has not been explored in the literature, except in the setting of cancer patients receiving cytotoxic chemotherapy, where it has been found to have no negative effects on clinical or psychological status of patients or their families and was cheaper than in-patient care (Mor *et al.* 1988b).

Cottage hospitals

Most of the studies of hospital palliative care have been based in teaching hospitals. Two papers draw attention to the role that small community hospitals can have in the provision of palliative care, particularly in rural areas (Seamark 1998, Johnson and Oliver 1991). In a retrospective survey comparing the terminal care of cancer patients in community hospitals and a hospice unit in western England, Seamark *et al.* (1998) found that hospice patients were more likely to be admitted for pain and symptom control, and less likely to be admitted for terminal nursing care than those admitted to community hospitals. Quantitatively, the care in the two settings was comparable, with the exception of poorer quality medical note keeping in community hospitals.

General strategies for improving terminal care in hospitals

Other possible strategies for improving the care of people dying in hospital are suggested in a number of studies, and include increased provision of single rooms (Walsh and Kingston 1988), facilities for carers who wish to remain close to a patient, particularly around the time of death (Walsh and Kingston 1988, Sykes *et al.* 1992), more undergraduate teaching to prepare student doctors (Ahmedzai 1982) and nurses (McWhan 1991) to care for dying patients, an examination of the impact of ward philosophies and prevailing inter-professional relationships on the nature of terminal care provided (Seale 1989, McWhan 1991, Mills *et al.* 1994), promotion of choice of place of death (Dunlop *et al.* 1989), and research to identify which patients benefit most from palliative care (Viney *et al.* 1994). Most of these reports were based on interview surveys of carers and hospital staff, and further research is needed in all these areas.

When both the consultant and senior nurse in a ward team showed caring characteristics the dying patient had more contact time and more attention from qualified nurses and received an acceptable standard of care. Teams in which the consultant withdrew from the patient and the senior nurse had a similar tendency showed a corresponding deficit in patient care. In these circumstances the care of dying patients, by default, became the responsibility of the junior nurse or an unqualified nursing assistant. . . .

Care extends beyond attention to physical needs: alleviation of individual patients' emotional, social, and spiritual problems should also be an integral part of their care. This requires that time be spent with patients to identify their needs. This requires a commitment to and a personal interst in the patients. As in other studies, this was rarely observed: contact between nurses and the dying patients was minimal; and distancing and isolation of patients were evident, the isolation increasing as death approached. ... (Mills *et al.* 1994)

Costs

The costs and benefits of various models of palliative care have already been discussed in question 4, and the limited information available on hospital services will only be outlined here.

The costs and nature of care delivered to terminally ill cancer patients in the acute hospital setting are explored in several American studies, in the context of the close link between definitions of 'hospice' and financial reimbursement. In the UCLA study discussed above, there were no significant differences in overall costs for hospice and control groups (Kane *et al.* 1984). Patton (1990) in a study conducted in a 44-bedded haematology–oncology nursing unit in Columbia. Where is this? found that a small subpopulation (0.8% of all admissions) of terminally ill cancer patients, funded by Medicare, accounted for high average lengths of stay, and their associated costs effectively eliminated terminal care profitability in the study year. To reduce costs he recommended the early identification of cancer patients in the terminal phase, more active involvement of hospitals in delivering long-term care, multidisciplinary case management, and hospice support. Whether these recommendations were implemented and proved cost effective is not reported. Hannan and O'Donnell (1984) compared three models of hospice programme in New York State: community-based, scattered-beds within a hospital, and an autonomous unit within a hospital. Four hospice programmes in each category were evaluated. They found that the charge per in-patient day was significantly higher for the hospital-based scattered-bed programmes, largely due to the increased diagnostic charges and room charges. However, there were large differences within each model as well, suggesting that differences were more dependent on local referral and operating policies than on inherent differences between the hospice models themselves.

Conclusion

To conclude, there is a paucity of research evaluating different models of palliative care provision within hospitals. The methodological issues involved in palliative care research, and discussed in chapter 5, are even more challenging in this setting, with a transient population of patients, under the care of a number of different teams, scattered throughout the hospital. Financial backing for such studies is frequently lacking. Services have developed to serve local need and resources, and the specifics of service provision must be taken into account in order to interpret evaluations meaningfully (Higginson and McCarthy 1989). This is well illustrated by previous discussion of the UCLA study (Kane *et al.* 1984).

The paper by Ellershaw *et al.* (1995). offers hope that hospital teams are rising to the challenge of evaluating their services. Evaluations of hospice units in the hospital setting, day hospitals, and the impact of clinical nurse specialists, are needed. However, wider issues need to be addressed to improve the care of those dying in hospital. The palliative care needs of those dying of non-malignant conditions particularly need to be considered. Educational initiatives to improve communication skills and pain and symptom control need to be described and evaluated. Research is also needed to identify which patients are most likely to benefit from palliative care, as well as investigating further the impact of ward philosophies and inter-professional relationships on the provision of terminal care.

Summary points

- Models of palliative care provision within hospitals have developed in response to local need and resources, and few services are directly comparable.
- The methodological challenges inherent in palliative care research are compounded in the hospital setting by the scattered and transient nature of the patient group.

- Few evaluative studies of hospital-based services are available, and it is not possible to make conclusive comments on the efficacy of any particular model.
- The hospital support team is currently the most popular model, and there is some evidence that it may be able to promote better symptom control, communication and liaison with community palliative care services at an earlier stage of illness than that available with conventional care alone.
- More research is needed on: the efficacy of in-patient palliative care units and day hospitals; the role of the clinical nurse specialist; palliative care of patients with non-malignant diagnoses; educational initiatives and the impact of ward philosophies. Both qualitative and quantitative approaches are needed.

Question 10 ....

Care for patients with cancer or other conditions

EMMA K. WILKINSON

What is the relationship between models of palliative care in cancer and models of palliative care in other diseases?

Focus of the research

The palliative care approach, which aims to promote both psychosocial and physical well-being, 'is a vital and integral part of all clinical practice, whatever the illness or its stage' (Wiles 1995). This section examines the extent to which this statement is borne out in practice. In other words, the extent to which the principles of palliative care are relevant in theory and applicable in practice to those dying of diseases other than cancer.

The articles reviewed for the section mainly consisted of non-experimental, expert opinion papers, or those which provided a description of care with no detailed data. There were relatively few papers which compared models of palliative care in cancer and palliative care for non-cancer diseases directly. In terms of the geographical spread of papers, most of the literature reviewed was based on research or expert opinion in the UK or North America.

Historical and social perspectives

Over the last two decades, palliative care for cancer patients has become well established and has expanded (Higginson 1993a). Research indicates that the typical hospice patient is a white male with terminal cancer (Mor and Masterson-Allen 1987). It would seem that a close association between the concepts 'cancer' and 'hospice' has been formed.

In spite of the key tenet of the palliative care approach to provide care to all patients regardless of disease or social setting (Wiles 1995), there is some evidence that attitudes towards cancer and non-cancer patients differ. Seale (1989) argues that the 'social meaning' of dying of cancer and dying of non-cancer differs and that this may, in turn, have an impact on treatment decisions and even fund-raising. Indeed, it is argued that cancer patients are seen as having a 'clearly delineated right of entry into the sick role', compared to non-cancer patients dying of terminal illness.

Survey work on consumer preferences and opinions has reflected such views. Public values expressed in surveys consistently indicate that moral judgements are made regarding healthcare for those whose suffering is perceived as self-inflicted, including, for example people with AIDS (Blaxter 1995). Consumer survey responses also show that the physically ill are consistently given priority over the mentally ill in terms of research priorities (Blaxter 1995). The impact of these widely held views on decision-making and priority setting is difficult to determine.

Provision of care

Little is known about the appropriate level of service provision required by people dying of causes other than cancer (Addington-Hall and McCarthy 1995b). The constantly changing physical symptoms characterized by most terminal non-cancer disorders (Doyle *et al.* 1993), as well as the changing needs of patients, are likely to contribute to the difficulty in planning palliative care.

A survey of palliative care services in Britain and Ireland in 1991 (Eve and Smith 1994) indicated that some palliative care programs for non-cancer patients, particularly for people with AIDS and motor neurone disease, have been established in the UK. Indeed, the survey indicated that of 139 in-patient units, just over 50% cared for patients with motor neurone disease, and almost as many cared for people with AIDS. Less than 4% said they would care for a patient with any terminal illness. In terms of the provision of day care, 64% of 129 day care units reported that they cared for patients with motor neurone disease, and 43% cared for people with AIDS. A significant number of day care unit would also care for other non-cancer patients, although exact details are not given. in the survey

163 hospital support teams were asked whether they would care only for cancer patients or whether patients with other diseases would be accepted. Of 52 hospital support teams that replied to this question, almost all would accept patients with motor neurone disease and AIDS. Almost two-thirds would accept patients with heart disease, or multiple sclerosis, and approximately a half would care for patients with Alzheimer's disease, strokes, or Parkinson's disease. Almost half said they would care for any terminally ill patient, and some specifically mentioned renal failure, diverticular disease, ischaemic problems, rheumatoid arthritis, and vascular disease. No evidence was given with regard to the actaul number of patients referred.

There was no literature which specifically focused on the provision of care in North America for people dying of causes other than cancer in the review.

Comparative research

There has been little research on the conditions and quality of 'non-hospice palliative care' received by cancer patients to provide any 'baseline measure' from which to compare the experiences of non-cancer patients (Seale 1989). An experimental study which specifically compared the experiences of 168 cancer patients to 471 'non-cancer' patients during the last year of life found several differences (Seale 1991c). Non-cancer patients were more likely to live alone or in a nursing home, and were less likely to receive help from families. Cancer patients were more likely to enter a hospice or hospital and were also more likely to know their diagnosis and prognosis. The deterioration of non-cancer patients tended to be more gradual, whereas cancer patients experienced more short-lived, intense pain. Non-cancer patients also experienced more problems with communication owing to their gradual deterioration and mental confusion, especially in the elderly. Also, non-cancer patients tended to be dependent on others for longer periods. Overall, cancer patients' predictable symptoms and better communication were more conducive to more effective planning of services.

As there are relatively few direct comparative studies examining the differences and similarities between cancer and non-cancer patients, the rest of this section examines the needs and provision of palliative care for specific, non-cancer diseases.

Terminal renal failure

The absence of literature on palliative care for patients dying of terminal renal failure was notable. Papers which did address this issue were mainly letters or papers outlining expert opinion and experimental papers were generally small scale.

In the USA, Oreopoulos (1995) argues that there is a need for better palliative care for patients who withdraw from dialysis, to ensure that their spiritual, psychological, and physical needs are met. It is further argued that a greater exchange of ideas between nephrologists and palliative experts may facilitate improvements in the provision of care. Some evidence for a need for improved palliation of symptoms was found by Cohen (1995) who examined the quality of death of 18 patients who died in a hospital unit or free-standing dialysis centre after the cessation of dialysis. A wide variation in survival rates was found between 2 and 34 days and death was not necessarily quick or painless for all patients. It was argued that improved palliative care could have ameliorated prolonged suffering, delirium and inadequately treated pain experienced by some patients.

In the UK, one paper indicated that adequate support for terminal renal patients' physical symptoms and psychosocial support in a hospice setting can be difficult to arrange (Andrews 1995). Indeed, the replies of 20 hospices and hospital-based palliative care units within the Thames Region to a questionnaire regarding referral indicated that 13 had never received an uncomplicated referral and were unwilling to accept patients for a variety of reasons. The main reasons for not accepting patients included: uncertain prognosis, fears of heavy workload, inexperience, and policy issues. However, 11 units had managed renal failure as a secondary diagnosis and of these a minority had managed the specific problems of renal disease: mycoclonic jerks, hallucinations, opioid sensitivity and emotional issues related to the stopping of dialysis. As such, it was argued the lack of receptivity of palliative care teams to accept patients is borne of unfamiliarity with the condition, rather than the lack of skills and knowledge to palliate the symptoms.

Motor neurone disease

A small number of papers addressed the needs and provision of palliative care for patients with motor neurone disease. Of these, most examined the role of in-patient hospice care for such patients within the UK (Saunders *et al.* 1981, O'Brien *et al.* 1992, Ellershaw 1993, Hicks and Corcoran 1993, Kelly and Cats 1994) and a few focused on the possibility of palliative care in the home (Moore 1993, Oliver 1996). The range of symptoms and symptomatic treatments as well as alleviation of psychosocial concerns are well documented in these papers. The lack of literature from North America on hospice type care for motor neurone disease patients may reflect the fact that care is still mainly reliant on informal care-givers (Norris 1992).

While some types of motor neurone disease are relatively benign, the most common is amyotrophic lateral sclerosis, which in its progression exacts a very severe toll, not only on the sufferer but usually on the family as well. ... These patients may live many months and even many years, so withholding supportive and symptomatic treatment adds appreciably to the duration of suffering. On the other hand, providing such treatment often increases the sufferer's quality of life in the remaining time. (Norris *et al.* 1985)

Hospices in the UK have become more involved in the care of patients in hospices and at home. Even though motor neurone disease is relatively rare, the wide range of symptoms in adult life are amenable to hospice care mainly because they are relatively predictable and manageable. However, survival rates vary (Saunders *et al.* 1981, O'Brien *et al.* 1992) and as symptoms often require active treatment from onset, hospice care is not a practical full-time option. Even so, intermittent hospice care has proved beneficial in providing an opportunity for respite care, the palliation of symptoms, rectifying problems in community care, and bereavement care (O'Brien *et al.* 1992, Hicks and Corcoran 1993, Kelly and Cats 1994). Uncontrolled pain and constipation have been the main symptoms which required palliation on referral (Saunders *et al.* 1981, O'Brien *et al.* 1992, Hicks and Corcoran 1993). Other common symptoms have included dysarthria, dysphagia, dypsnoea, insomnia, fatigue, and incontinence (Saunders *et al.* 1981). There is thus a broad scope for symptom control. The use of opiates within the hospice environment at the terminal phase has proved to be a safe and effective option in the palliation of symptoms (Norris *et al.* 1985). Despite the availability of symptomatic treatments, some argue that the alleviation of symptoms is still inadequate (Norris 1992). In the final stage of the disease deterioration is usually rapid (O'Brien *et al.* 1992), although this is not always the case.

The complexity of caring for patients with motor neurone disease involves the alleviation of psychosocial concerns as well as physical symptoms. For example, mood swings, depression and anxiety (Hicks and Corcoran 1993, Kelly and Cats 1994), and fear of choking to death (Kelly and Cats 1994) are common amongst motor neurone disease patients. Psychosocial concerns of the family may include the emotional strain of caring for relatives on a long-term basis (Kelly and Cats 1994), the shock of sudden deterioration which may occur before death (Ellershaw 1993) or the problems associated with the patients' gradual loss of speech. The use of aids may improve the patients' quality of life and may also help to alleviate some psychosocial problems by facilitating better communication as well as the promotion of comfort (Ellershaw 1993).

Palliative care at home for motor neurone disease patients has become a potential option for some patients in the UK and US. It has been suggested that palliative care at home is a preferable option for most patients whose cognitive functioning remains intact during the progression of the disease and who are motivated to stay in control of as much of their lives as possible (Moore 1993). In general, home care is only made possible through a collaborative effort based on the co-ordination of specialist health professionals, informal carers, and voluntary groups (Moore 1993, Oliver 1996). The home care option is not open to all patients, especially those without a live-in carer.

Terminal cardiovascular disease

There is relatively little literature on models of palliative care for those dying of terminal cardiovascular disease or stroke. No papers addressed such issues in North America, with the exception of the SUPPORT trial (Study to Understand Prognoses and Preferences for Outcomes and Risks of Treatment, Connors *et al.* 1995). In the UK, until recently, the literature has addressed the issue of the lack of provision of care and reasons why palliative care may not be applicable for such patients. These papers have been based on expert opinion. Indeed, Jones (1995) has argued that there is little research into the possible benefits of hospice care for patients dying of cardiac failure, and that this is may be due to the lack of recognition of the poor prognosis of such patients. Similarly, others have argued for the need for better palliation of symptoms such as dypsnoea, tiredness, and cachexia (Cushen 1994) especially as symptomatic treatments exist such as the use of low-dose opiates to ease dyspnoea. Speculation regarding the lack of palliative care services has centred on the relatively small numbers of patients that receive palliative care and the considerable demands which these patients place on services (Beattie 1995).

... many patients who die of stroke do not receive optimal symptom control or sufficient help to overcome psychological morbidity. Their informal care-givers experience difficulty in getting the information they need about the patient's medical condition. ... Taken together, they demonstrate the importance of providing care for stroke patients and their families that encompasses their physical, emotional, and social needs and aims to improve the quality of life remaining. (Addington-Hall *et al.* 1995)

More recently, several experimental studies have focused on the quality of care experienced by patients and carers in non-hospice environments (Addington-Hall *et al.* 1995, McCarthy *et al.* 1996, McCarthy *et al.* 1997b). The results suggest that there is room for improvement with regard to the physical aspects of care. Addington-Hall *et al.* (1995) examined the quality of care received by a representative sample of 237 patients in general hospital across 20 health districts during their last year of life. of these patients 65% had experienced pain, which was only partially alleviated in 50% of cases. Over half the patients also experienced low mood and urinary incontinence. Similar findings were outlined in an interview survey of 600 informal care-givers on the quality of life of stroke patients in their last year of life (McCarthy *et al.* 1996). Symptom control was limited in general hospitals, and over half the patients experienced pain, dyspnoea and low mood. Some symptoms were found to be distressing, including faecal incontinence, mood, anxiety, pain, nausea and mental confusion, and some symptoms lasted for more than 6 months.

These surveys also highlighted the need for improved psychosocial support for families (Addington-Hall *et al.* 1995), more information (Addington-Hall *et al.* 1995) and more patient choice on treatment decisions (McCarthy *et al.* 1996). Communication between health professionals and stroke patients and families in terms of prognoses was found to be inadequate (McCarthy *et al.* 1997b). These authors also found that only 26% of a representative sample of 600 patients across 20 health districts reported that they knew they were likely to die and of these, the majority had worked this out alone. Also, 43% of informal care-givers felt that they had had insufficient choice in terms of the place of death and 63% would have liked to have been present at death.

Dementia/Alzheimer's disease

The prevalence of dementia in Europe indicates that the incidence of dementia in those aged between 60 and 65 is approximately 1% and this nearly doubles with every 5 year increase in age from the ages of 60 to 94 (Hofman *et al.* 1991). Under the age of 75 there is a higher prevalence of dementia in men compared to women, although this is reversed after the age of 75 (Hofman *et al.* 1991). The fact that patients dying of dementia or Alzheimer's are mainly elderly has particular relevance to the application of palliative care principles. Differences in the incidence, duration, intensity, and type of symptoms experienced by elderly patients with multiple diagnoses and multisystem pathology, compared to most terminal cancer patients, underscores the need for a different type of palliative care (Seale 1991c). Practical issues, such as ensuring adequate home care during the patients' illness, may be of more importance given the reduced social networks of elderly patients. On the other hand, bereavement support of those left behind after the death of the patient, is less frequently required owing to reduced social networks. Difficulties in achieving open communication between carer and patient may occur.

Knowledge about the terminal care preferences of decisionally impaired patients is frequently unavailable, and therefore, it is often necessary for families and professional caregivers to make surrogate judgments as to the kind of terminal care the patient should receive. (Hanrahan and Luchins 1993)

Relatively few research studies have investigated the needs, experience or provision of care for people dying of dementia/Alzheimer's in the UK. However, a recent, comparative retrospective study, drawn from the Regional Study of Care for the Dying, addressed these issues (McCarthy *et al.* 1997a). These authors examined the experiences of 1513 cancer patients who had received hospice care, compared to 170 dementia patients. The results showed that although the symptoms experienced by both groups were similar, those of the dementia patients were longer in duration. Dementia patients had a greater need for home care and they received more home help and residential care than their cancer counterparts, although they also received less general practitioner and nursing care. Over a third of informal carers of dementia patients complained about the lack of peace and quiet in hospitals. In terms of the impact on the family, 35% of informal carers of dementia patients found the care rewarding, compared to 60% of carers of cancer patients. Dementia carers also suffered less adverse affects of bereavement. Another study, which examined the most prevalent symptoms during the terminal phase of 17 patients receiving care in psychogeriatric wards, found that dyspnoea, pain, and pyrexia were most common and that most patients were polysymptomatic (Lloyd-Williams 1996b). Furthermore, the notes indicated that all patients were in distress during the last 48–72 hours and that the opioid prescribing was erratic. These studies indicate that there is room for improvement in the palliative care of people with dying from dementia in the UK, as well as a need for more research into how best their needs can be met.

Most of the literature in North America has focused on ways to accurately predict survival time, rather than specific aspects of palliative care (Thal 1993, Volicer 1993, Maletta 1995) as a result of the Medicare financial reimbursement scheme which requires patients to have a life expectancy of 6 months or less. Similar research has also focused on potential adjustments to the current hospice admission criteria (Hanrahan and Luchins 1995b). The goal of this research is to improve the availability and access to hospice care for end-stage dementia patients. Difficulties in gaining access to hospice care are highlighted by some studies. A questionnaire survey given to 1184 hospice directors indicated that in 1990, fewer than 1% of hospice patients had a primary diagnosis of severe dementia with no concurrent diagnosis, although 7% of patients had dementia as a secondary diagnosis to another terminal illness. According to Hanrahan and Luchins (1995a) the general reluctance of hospices to admit end-stage dementia patients was due to difficulties in predicting survival time, the need of patients' families for respite care which may exceed the constraints of the care program, and the need for more staff training to care for dementia patients. As well as problems with the accessibility of hospice care, Collins and Ogle (1994) argue that long-term institutional care is also not meeting the needs of patients, as much care is reliant on informal care-givers in the home. However, more research is required to affirm whether this is a reliable conclusion.

Given the practical, and potential ethical problems, of integrating the hospice care of cancer patients and end-stage dementia patients, the provision of specialized, segregated in-patient units has been made available to some patients (Hurley *et al.* 1993, Wilson *et al.* 1996). One such programme described by Wilson *et al.* (1996), which involves a cluster of special hospice units linked to long-term nursing homes, differs from traditional hospice cancer care in several ways. The interventions are less pharmacologic than those provided to typical cancer hospice patients, and there is less emphasis on alleviating nausea and pain, and more emphasis on psychosocial care.

Other research in North America has focused on the decision-making process behind choosing the most appropriate management or type of care for end-stage dementia patients (Volicer *et al.* 1986, Luchins and Hanrahan 1993, Pfeiffer 1995). This is seen as a key aspect of care as patients are unable to communicate their own views, so the most ethical way of deciding how to care for them most appropriately is paramount for carers and health professionals. Volicer (1986) proposed a model of care in which health professionals and families chose one of five levels of care, ranging from aggressive to purely supportive care, depending on the condition of the patient. The underlying aim was to maximize comfort through the use of analgesics and oxygen, but not to prolong suffering. However, Enck (1987) argues that clinical situations are not so clear-cut and that an individual approach to meeting patients' needs is more appropriate.

HIV and AIDS

The growth of literature in both the UK and North America illustrates the recognized importance of applying the principles of palliative care to those suffering from HIV/AIDS.

Common features of advanced HIV/AIDS which are likely to differ from advanced cancer include the predominantly younger age group, the treatments such as blood transfusions and intravenous therapies given to maintain quality of life, homelessness or inadequate housing, the difficulty in identifying a terminal phase and the more complex relations with family and friends. Many symptoms and the need for total care are similar, however, and it would seem sensible to adapt or expand palliative services to include people with HIV/AIDS. (Higginson 1993a)

The diverse physical and psychosocial needs of people with HIV/AIDS are well documented in the literature. The various stages of the disease are not clear-cut and there is rarely a clear transition from active, aggressive treatment to palliative care. Aggressive treatment to control disease progression and symptoms may continue until death. Common symptoms in advanced HIV include chronic fatigue, neurological problems such as blindness, dementia, multiple infections, weakness, diarrhoea, muscle wasting, and dyspnoea. The nature of symptoms may change in number and severity with the disease progression, making frequent review necessary (Walsh 1991). These fluctuations in clinical condition make the terminal phase itself more difficult to define (McKeogh 1995). In general, the person with advanced HIV infection has a wider variety of medical problems than someone with terminal cancer. Rapid advances in treatment make prognosis difficult to determine, and the nature of patients' problems may change.

On a social level, the needs of people with HIV/AIDS also differ, in some ways, from those of people with terminal cancer. People with HIV/AIDS tend to be younger, more vocal, and more autonomous than patients with terminal cancer (Mansfield *et al*. 1992). Having a life-threatening illness at this stage of life often leads to a re-assessment of life goals. Often people with HIV/AIDS lack financial security. Problems in funding healthcare, as well as ensuring adequate housing, are common practical concerns. As well as living with the psychosocial impact of their own symptoms and fear of the future, they also have to contend with complex societal prejudices. Furthermore, those with HIV/AIDS may have more complicated relationships, in which informal carers themselves may be infected. Patients may not want to inform family of their illness, and carers are less likely to be family members. The difference in the pattern of illness, the wider range of physical needs and the more complicated social issues have led to a different application of palliative care principles for people with HIV/AIDS.

In the UK, community-based models of care have been established and in general, are geographically based in accordance with the prevalence of HIV/AIDS. The increase in palliative services within the community is due to the increasing pressure on hospital beds, economic incentives and is also driven by patient and carer preference for care at home (Johnson 1989). The growth in the number of special outreach teams, especially in London, reflects this trend. These teams provide practical medical help, as well as advice and psychosocial support, and aim to provide links with other care available in the community and bereavement support (Butters *et al.* 1991, McCann 1991).

Even though specialist outreach teams compare favourably with other community services from a patient and carer perspective (Higginson *et al.* 1990, McCann 1991, Butters *et al.* 1993), recent studies indicate that there is still some room for improvement. For example, a study of 140 people with HIV/AIDS receiving home palliative care from outreach teams in an inner city area found that symptom control was a commonly severe problem at referral and remained a common problem throughout care. Weakness, diarrhoea, muscle wasting, memory loss, visual problems, and dyspnoea proved the most difficult symptoms for the team to alleviate, especially in the last week of care. Patient anxiety and pain levels although initially high, were substantially reduced (Butters *et al.* 1992). McCann and Hadsworth (1992) found some evidence that the physical and emotional needs of informal care-givers of people with AIDS were not being met adequately. Of 125 informal care-givers interviewed, 70% believed they gave both practical and emotional support to the patient and approximately one third would have liked more help themselves with this care. Only 42% felt that the home care team provided care only for the patient. Another study indicated that although care provided by primary care and hospital teams was generally successful in facilitating care in the community, a greater emphasis on social support and counselling was advocated (Smits *et al.* 1990)

The statutory services within the community have been complemented by voluntary groups (Anonymous 1989, Partridge 1989, Singh 1989, Thomson 1989). Voluntary groups play a key a role in addressing the needs of minority groups, including children or women with HIV/AIDS, drug users, those with HIV/AIDS in prison, and those who have haemophilia as well as HIV/AIDS. According to Cranfield (1989) housing needs, as well as isolation are paramount concerns of drug users with HIV/AIDS. This is because services for these people are mainly based in inner city areas, and treatment of symptoms requires moving to an area where housing is difficult to obtain, especially for drug users. Some practical measures in addressing these needs have been taken by some voluntary groups, e.g. by the Terrence Higgins Trust. Overall, relatively few experimental studies have examined the needs and service provision of minority groups and as such, it is difficult to determine the extent to which their needs are being met.

In North America, some of the literature has focused on similar psychosocial issues and the diverse needs of people with HIV/AIDS (Gilmore 1987, Anonymous 1988a, Kemp and Stepp 1995). These are mainly opinion papers; relatively few are experimental. The findings suggest that needs are similar, especially in suburban areas, where models of care have to attempt to meet problems of homelessness, confidentiality, housing, and transportation (Martin 1986, McCann 1991). In terms of psychosocial needs, a comparison of hospice patients with AIDS, compared to those with other diagnoses, indicated that people with AIDS were significantly less likely to receive social support than those with other diagnoses and also required more psychosocial support. Hospice staff felt that working with people with AIDS was more time-consuming and stressful than working with non-AIDS patients due to the diverse physical and emotional needs, as well as the unpredictable course of the disease trajectory (Baker and Seager 1991).

Much of the literature focused on the quality of care provided by the various models of hospice care. Several, non-experimental, opinion papers have proposed models of care (Schofferman 1987, Martin 1988) or have described the development of hospice programs (Martin 1986). Other research has focused on the difficulties in planning care for patients whose disease is unpredictable (Clark *et al.* 1988), and whether hospice staff may lack the appropriate skills to care for people with HIV/AIDS (Stephany 1992). The complexity and diversity of need in the context of a hospice environment has also been examined. For example, a comparative study of hospice care for 143 people with AIDS, compared to 120 Medicare patients, indicated that people with AIDS were twice as likely to be hospitalized during their hospital stay, consumed more drugs in the hospice, and required skilled therapy and attendant care services more frequently. Some have argued that, in spite of the complexity of care needs, resources are not being adequately channelled into hospice programs to meet these needs (Kovacs and Rodgers 1995). These authors found that although 85% of 148 hospice directors indicated that their hospices were serving people with HIV/AIDS, only 9% had hired extra staff to meet their needs.

Less research has addressed the role of secondary care centres in the community (Goldstone 1992, Goldstone *et al.* 1995). Goldstone (1992) examined the trends of hospital utilization between 1987 and 1991 in a teaching hospital and found that hospitals were still playing a major role in their terminal care, and this was linked to the fact that less patients were able to die at home owing to carer exhaustion and the longer life-span which was associated with a wider range of symptoms. However, it was argued that better symptom management, more chronic palliative care beds, and higher staffing levels were required to meet the diverse needs of patients. Overall, the general lack of research into the provision of care within the community makes it difficult to draw firm conclusions regarding the extent to which palliative care is meeting the needs of people with HIV/AIDS in North America,.

Other non-cancer diseases

Virtually no literature addressed the potential relevance or applicability of the principles of palliative care for terminally ill patients dying from chronic respiratory disesease, progressive neurological diseases such as multiple sclerosis or Parkinson's disease, or neuromuscular disorders such as cerebral palsy, Duchenne's muscular dystrophy, or spinal muscle atrophy. The reasons for the lack of literature are not clear.

There is some evidence that the adoption of the palliative care approach may be appropriate in addressing the physical and psychosocial concerns of those dying from these incurable diseases. In general, the application of appropriate palliative care techniques early on can improve the clinical disability and may hinder the disease progression of those suffering from neurological diseases

(Obbens 1997). The reduction of pain can also improve quality of life. This is especially true of those people with multiple sclerosis for whom pain can occur at any stage of the disease (Payne and Gonzales 1997), as well as those with rheumatoid arthritis (Galasko 1997). The impact of some of these neurological diseases or incurable orthopeadic conditions can be devastating, and the principles of palliative care are appropriate in addressing the patients' needs. For example, the increasing sense of isolation and negative body image experienced by some people dying of chronic obstructive pulmonary disease (COPD) as they gradually become inactive should not be overlooked by those responsible for their care (Shee 1995).

Conclusion

The scarcity of literature on the relevance of palliative care for non-cancer patients was notable, especially for patients suffering from renal failure, motor neurone disease, or dementia/Alzheimer's. Reasons for this lack of literature are not fully understood, and it is difficult to determine, on the basis of this literature, whether the needs of such patients are being met and whether they have access to appropriate care. The recent experimental work on palliative care for terminal cardiovascular disease has provided firmer evidence for a need for more respect for choice and autonomy in the palliative care provided in hospitals as well as more attention to symptom control. The research on HIV/AIDS is generally more substantive and interest in addressing the needs of people with AIDS has grown substantially in the last decade, although the extent to which care is meeting these needs is more difficult to determine from the literature.

From an ethical perspective, the provision of palliative care for all patients, regardless of disease or social context, is indisputable. In practice, the application of the principles of palliative care has proved difficult in many cases. This is partially the result of rarity of some terminal diseases, which affect only a small number of patients, or the difficulty in predicting life expectancy in the case of heart disease, stroke and renal disease. The planning of care for such patients has proved problematic. On a practical level, adapting the care environments initially set up for terminal cancer patients can prove to be time-consuming and costly, especially for patients requiring special aids or equipment, such as motor neurone disease patients. Also, the diversity of symptoms experienced by some patients may require a different approach to the provision of care, although the underlying principles of palliative care remain relevant. Furthermore, the unpredictable nature of most non-cancer diseases means that addressing the spiritual, physical, and psychological aspects of care over the entire duration over their terminal illness may prove both impractical and impossible due to the limited capacity and resources of programs of palliative care. Clearly, more research is required to examine further the extent to which the diverse needs of terminally ill non-cancer patients are being met, in all care settings, in both the UK and North America.

III

Conclusions

Implications of the findings for the health services

NICK BOSANQUET

The main conclusions of our review are positive: a new kind of care has developed and has led to results for many thousands of patients. There is a significant new resource in knowledge and skill of staff. This programme has also been a significant example of a different kind of innovation—not one which started with large research programmes or in the prestigous medical establishments, but one which began with a few concerned individuals using voluntary rather than government funding. In its further development the programme challenges conventional stereotypes of UK and US healthcare with palliative care developing in the US on a low cost community base away from the large hospitals in a kind of programme more often associated with the UK.

For the future there will be significant changes in the context within which palliative care will develop:

- As populations age, a larger proportion of healthcare will be palliative care for older people. A model which was originally developed for younger patients with cancer will now have to adapt to many older patients and to a wider range of diagnoses.

- The boundaries between palliative care and care of long-term chronic illness are likely to change. The challenge of palliative care will be that of reducing disability as well as of providing terminal care.

- There will be a continuing shift of care towards a home and community base. This will be driven by three main forces:
  - patient and carer demand
  - new technology and informatics which will make it much more possible to develop personal care programmes and to monitor results
  - pressures from the reduced availability of long-term care.

- Even if the number of nursing home places does not reduce further in absolute terms there will be fewer places in relation to past measures of need. Thus there will be more frail elderly people living in the community.
- Palliative care will have to face more questions about value as funding constraints increase and as the range of potential investments widen.

The aim can be a highly positive one—that of securing quality of life and freedom from pain during the last phase. Palliative care holds out the promise of a period before death which could be lived free from pain, with dignity protected and last opportunities for positive experience. Such an aim is feasible with current drug therapy and the current state of knowledge on pain control. It is not a far-off dream, but an aim which could be achieved at reasonable cost using known therapies and techniques. Yet no country in the world, even those which have made the most investment in palliative care, is close to achieving this goal. Rather the situation is one in which many patients face pain, great anxiety, and loss of dignity in the last period of life. The take-up of palliative care has been patchy between countries, with virtually no interest in most of Europe outside the UK and Italy: but it has also been patchy within countries. The results in terms of achieved outcomes for all potential patients from investment in palliative care have been disappointing.

There is a major development challenge facing palliative care in the next phase: how to meet higher expectations for evidence-based effective care, how to win friends and achieve results in a world of rising constraints and possibly of greater scepticism. Palliative care will be expected to provide a more flexible, home-based service to a greater range of groups. It will operate under greater funding constraints and it will have to make choices about the types of project and service which are to be funded. It is also likely that specialist palliative care will be playing a complementary role to non-specialist care. Most palliative care will be given by non-specialists. For the UK there will be new challenges in delivering palliative care within the new structure for cancer care. Within the US, oncologists are showing greater interest in palliative care.

Although there are pressures and challenges facing palliative care there are also strengths and opportunities in terms of experience in organizing services, a high level of teamwork and a well-established international community.

Against this background we have reviewed research on service patterns, needs, models of organization, consumers' views, and other topics. We would signal some concern about the standard and relevance of work done over the past 10 years. When the service faced the challenge of becoming established at all there was a greater willingness to commission work on a comparative and probing basis. The first generation of work done in the 1970s and early 1980s was more ambitious than much of the recent work, which has often been rather descriptive and of local and short-term interest. There are few robust results and established findings to guide decisions about funding or the management of services. The field of palliative care is still to a great extent guided by general sentiment rather than specifically tested insights into how to develop more effective services. However, we do not underestimate the costs and difficulties involved in conducting robust and generalizable evaluations.

Although the difficulties of conducting research in palliative care have been discussed, it should be possible to conduct rigorous randomized trials, for example by randomizing patients by general practice or by district, rather than by the individual patient. Such large studies will be extremely expensive to conduct, but this may be cost-effective in the context of the national investment in specialist palliative care, and the remaining uncertainties about the benefits of different models of organization.

Our results have practical implications for healthcare. Palliative care is sometimes seen as a rather well-defined area with little change or new process. It should instead be seen as a field which is subject to many new stresses and to new problems of delivering care. Our central message is that research needs to contribute to a more active development process in palliative care, which should be seen as a field in which better results are only going to come about through a willingness to look for new solutions.

We want to see a research agenda which will generate information for a new phase of creative development. We would see the focus as being much more on specific areas of client groups and policy issues. Research on the very general area of palliative care is likely to be less rewarding than in the past. Within this context of the search for change in local process, research needs to explore options, define choices and provide more evidence on trade-offs. It also needs to find ways of making it possible to collect patient and carer views at the local level. There is a particular dearth of information for example about their experience with non-specialist care.

Key areas include changing and broadening in patient groups; new challenges in improving therapy; and the evaluation of différent models of care. Within this framework, some examples of topics could be as follows:

- Changing patient 'need':
  - the palliative care needs of patients with non-cancer diagnoses
  - the implications of change in oncology for palliative care needs of patients with cancer
  - options for improving palliative care in nursing homes and long-term care.
- New challenges in therapy
  - the positive use of drug therapy in palliative care: there is very little research on drug therapy/prescribing decisions in palliative care.
  - improving communication with carers.
  - the development of psychosocial counselling and support as part of palliative care.

Models of care

There remain some very important questions which have been addressed by innumerable small descriptive studies with inconclusive results of limited generalizability. There is still a need for well-conducted large scale studies to provide strong evidence on the following issues:

- Whether or not home palliative care support teams and hospital support teams improve quality of life, symptom control, or any other aspects of care other than patient satisfaction.
- The cost-effectiveness of in-patient palliative care in free-standing hospices in comparison with conventional hospital care and intensive home care support.
- Alternative approaches to the development of skills and communication in teams in palliative care. We would also wish to see

support for more research into the perceptions and concerns of staff.

- The development of teams and shared process between primary and secondary care.
- The role of volunteers and self-help groups.
- The role of day hospitals.
- The costs and benefits arising from the clinical nurse specialist role in hospital.
- The different roles of family doctors or primary care physicians in palliative care and different ways of improving their ability to care.

For the future, palliative care will be a network where human capital in skill and knowledge will often be more crucial than buildings. The role of hospices will change and evolve and the spirit of the hospice will take different service forms. The aim is a vital one—a network providing an accessible, effective service to all those who need it in a local community. Palliative care will move to a process of further local achievement. A new set of challenges now has to be faced. Palliative care could be one of the most positive areas of care development in the next two decades.

Palliative care has developed through a strong sense of specialist mission. It may well be difficult to share this mission with a wider audience, yet the gains in patients' quality of life could be great. Past investment in palliative care has created a valuable resource that is now local rather than exceptional, but there will be more pressure to demonstrate value for money. The challenge in different ways, both in the US and the UK, is how to use this resource so that all patients, including those with non-cancer diagnoses, can benefit from access to better care. In an era of financial constraints, new alliances are needed for shared care if the full promise of palliative care is to be realized.

Appendices

Appendix A
Organizations contacted for details of unpublished work or on-going research

Association for Palliative Medicine of Great Britain and Ireland, Association of Cancer Physicians, British Association for Cancer Research, British Association of Surgical Oncology, British Medical Association, British Oncology Association, Cancer Relief Macmillan Fund, Cancer Research Campaign, Department of Health, Imperial Cancer Research Fund, Institute of Cancer Research, Leukaemia Research Fund, Marie Curie Cancer Care, Medical Research Council, Royal College of General Practitioners, Royal College of Nursing, Royal College of Physicians, Royal College of Surgeons of England, Royal Marsden Hospital, The Cochrane Collaboration, The National Cancer Alliance, UK Children's Cancer Study Group, UK Co-ordinating Committee on Cancer Research, Wellcome Trust

Appendix B
Individuals approached to provide bibliographies or details of work in progress

Dr Julia Addington-Hall, Dr Sam Ahmedzai, Dr J.C. Bass, Mrs I Bezic, Miss L Bycroft, Dr D Clark, Mrs S Duke, Professor A Faulkner, Dr David Field, Dr Marilene Filbet, Professor Barry Hancock, Professor Irene Higginson, Dr L Hockey, Dr Ian Johnson, Dr Peter Leiberich, Dr Mark McCarthy, Ms E.R. McKee, Dr Hans Moolenburgh, Ms J Mulligan, Mrs M Mullins, Dr Brenda Neale, Dr B Noble, Dr Marilyn Relf, Dr Julia Riley, Dr D Seamark, Dr Bruce Sizer, Mrs Carol Stone, Dr F Toscani, Dr H.W. van den Borne, Professor Eric Wilkes, Mrs H Woolley

Appendix C
General search strategy

1 explode 'PALLIATIVE-CARE'/ all subheadings

2 explode 'TERMINAL-CARE'/ all subheadings

3 'HOSPICES' OR 'HOSPICE-CARE'/ all subheadings

4 explode 'ONCOLOGIC-NURSING'/ all subheadings

5 explode 'CANCER-CARE-FACILITIES'/ all subheadings

6 #1 or #2 or #3 or #4 or #5

7 #6 and ((NURS* OR CARER* OR CARING OR HOSPI* OR TEAM* OR DEATH OR DYING OR SERVICE* OR NEED* OR DEMAND* OR FAMIL* OR HEALTH OR POLICY OR MODEL* OR DELIVERY OR EVALUAT* OR PROGRAM* OR UTILI?A-TION OR ORGANI?ATION or HOME or PREFERENCE* OR CO?ORDINAT* OR EFFECT* OR ROLE OR QUALITY OR SUPPORT OR AUDIT) in TI)

8 'HOSPICES'/ economics , manpower , organization-and-admin-istration , supply-and-distribution , statistics-and-numerical-data , standards , trends , utilization

9 'TERMINAL-CARE'/ economics , manpower , organization-and-administration , supply-and-distribution , statistics-and-numer-ical-data , standards , trends , utilization

10 'PALLIATIVE-CARE'/ economics , manpower , organization-and-administration , supply-and-distribution , statistics-and-numer-ical-data , standards , trends , utilization

11 #7 OR #8 OR #9 OR #10

12 'DRUG-EVALUATION'/ all subheadings

13 explode 'DRUG-THERAPY'/ all subheadings

14 #11 not (#12 or #13)

15 #14 and ((LA='ENGLISH') OR (LA='FRENCH') OR (LA= 'GERMAN') OR (LA='ITALIAN') OR (LA='SWEDISH'))

16 #15 not ((RADIOTHERAPY or CHEMOTHERAPY or SURGERY) in TI,MESH)

17 #16 and (PY > '1979')

18 'CLINICAL-TRIALS'/ all subheadings

19 'CONTROLLED-CLINICAL-TRIALS'/ all subheadings

20 'MULTICENTER-STUDIES'/ all subheadings

21 explode 'RANDOMIZED-CONTROLLED-TRIALS'/ all sub-headings

22 explode 'NURSING-RESEARCH'/ ALL SUBHEADINGS

23 'PROGRAM-EVALUATION'/ ALL SUBHEADINGS

24 'EVALUATION-STUDIES'

25 explode 'HEALTH-SERVICES-RESEARCH'/ ALL SUBHEAD-INGS

26 'HEALTH-SURVEYS'

27 explode 'REVIEW-LITERATURE'/ all subheadings

28 'META-ANALYSIS'

29 explode 'QUESTIONNAIRES'/ all subheadings

30 'PATIENT-SATISFACTION' or 'CONSUMER-SATISFAC-TION'

31 'COST-BENEFIT-ANALYSIS'/ all subheadings

32 'OUTCOME-ASSESSMENT-HEALTH-CARE' or 'OUT-COME-AND-PROCESS-ASSESSMENT-HEALTH-CARE' OR 'HEALTH-SERVICES-NEEDS-AND-DEMAND'

33 (RANDOM* NEAR TRIAL*) IN TI

34 RANDOMIZED-CONTROLLED-TRIAL IN PT

35 META-ANALYSIS IN PT

36 CONTROLLED-CLINICAL-TRIAL IN PT

37 REVIEW-LITERATURE IN PT

38 #18 OR #19 OR #20 OR #21 OR #22 OR #23 OR #24 OR #25 OR #26 OR #27 OR #28 OR #29 OR #30 OR #31 OR #32 OR #33 OR #34 OR #35 OR #36 OR #37

39 #17 AND #38

This strategy identifies references which:

• have **any** of the main relevant palliative care Mesh headings

• **and** one of a number of key words; **or** one of the relevant Mesh subheadings

• **and** one of a number of relevant methodology types

- **and** meeting the date and language criteria
- but **excluding** studies concerned with drug evaluation, chemo-therapy, radiotherapy or surgery.

In addition to the above general strategy various further searches were performed for each research question. For example, searches for Question 7 included the use of terms relating to palliative care or terminal care combined with terms related to quality of life.

Appendix D
Checklists of quality of studies*

General checklist

Study design

Is the objective of the study sufficiently described?	Yes	Unclear	No
Was the design of the study appropriate to the objective?	Yes	Unclear	No
Is the source of the subjects clearly described?	Yes	Unclear	No
Is the method of selection of the subjects clearly described (i.e. inclusion and exclusion criteria)?	Yes	Unclear	No
Was the sample of subjects appropriate with regard to the population to which the findings will be referred?	Yes	Unclear	No
Was the sample size based on pre-study considerations of statistical power?	Yes	Unclear	No
Were the models of care/interventions well defined?	Yes	Unclear	No
Are the outcome measures appropriate?	Yes	Unclear	No

Conduct of study

Was a satisfactory (>60%) response rate achieved?	Yes	Unclear	No

---

* Based on checklists published by the NHS Centre for Reviews and Dissemination (1996) and by Altman (1991)

Analysis and presentation

Is there a statement adequately describing or referencing all the statistical procedures used?	Yes	Unclear	No
Were the statistical methods used appropriate for the data?	Yes	Unclear	No

Overall assessment

Are the conclusions drawn from the statistical analyses justified?	Yes	Unclear	No

Randomized controlled trials

Was the assignment to the treatment groups really random?	Yes	Unclear	No
Was randomization of the participants blinded?	Yes	Unclear	No
Was relatively complete follow-up achieved?	Yes	Unclear	No
Were the outcomes of people who withdrew described and included in the analysis?	Yes	Unclear	No
Were those assessing outcomes blind to the treatment allocation?	Yes	Unclear	No
Were the control and treatment groups comparable at entry?	Yes	Unclear	No
Were the groups treated identically other than for the named interventions?	Yes	Unclear	No

Cohort studies

Are the exposed people representative of the standard users of the intervention?	Yes	Unclear	No
Was the non-exposed cohort selected from the same population as the exposed?	Yes	Unclear	No
Were the cohorts comparable on any important confounding factors?	Yes	Unclear	No
Was there adequate adjustment for the effects of these confounding variables?	Yes	Unclear	No

Was outcome assessment blind to exposure status?	Yes	Unclear	No
Was follow-up long enough for the outcomes to occur?	Yes	Unclear	No
Was an adequate proportion of the cohort followed-up?	Yes	Unclear	No
Were drop-out rates similar in exposed and unexposed groups?	Yes	Unclear	No

Case–control studies

Has the disease state of the cases been reliably assessed and validated?	Yes	Unclear	No
Are the cases representative of a series, or is there a potential for selection bias?	Yes	Unclear	No
Were the controls selected from a similar population as the cases?	Yes	Unclear	No
Is there evidence that the controls are free from disease?	Yes	Unclear	No
How comparable are the cases and controls with respect to potential confounding factors?	Yes	Unclear	No
Were hazards and interventions assessed in the same way for cases and controls?	Yes	Unclear	No
Was the response rate adequate?	Yes	Unclear	No
Were the non-response rates the same in both groups?	Yes	Unclear	No
Is it possible that over-matching has occurred in that cases and controls were matched on factors related to exposure?	Yes	Unclear	No
Was an appropriate statistical analysis used (matched or unmatched)?	Yes	Unclear	No

Longitudinal surveys or case series

Is the study based on a random sample selected from a suitable sampling frame?	Yes	Unclear	No

Is there any evidence that the sample is
representative of standard users of the
intervention?   Yes Unclear No

Are the criteria for inclusion in the sample
clearly defined?   Yes Unclear No

Did all individuals enter the survey at a similar
point in their disease progression?   Yes Unclear No

Was follow-up long enough for important
events to occur?   Yes Unclear No

Were outcomes assessed using objective
criteria?   Yes Unclear No

If comparisons of series are being made, was
there sufficient description of the series and
the distribution of prognostic factors?   Yes Unclear No

Bibliography

The bibliography lists all the publications on which the review is based. Not all are referred to specifically in the text.

Aaronson, N.K. (1991) Methodologic issues in assessing the quality of life in cancer patients. *Cancer* 67, 844–50.

Abel, E.K. (1986) The hospice movement: Institutionalizing innovation. *Int J Health Serv* 16, 71–85.

Addington-Hall, J.M. (1996) Heart disease and stroke: lessons from cancer care. In Ford, G. and Lewin, I. (eds) *Interfaces in Medicine: managing terminal illness*. London: Royal College of Physicians.

Addington-Hall, J.M. and McCarthy, M. (1992). The regional study of care for the dying: a preliminary analysis of results by districts for the King's Fund Centre Conference 8 July 1992. Department of Epidemiology and Public Health, University College London.

Addington-Hall, J.M. and McCarthy, M. (1995a) Dying from cancer: results of a national population-based investigation. *Palliat Med* 9, 295–305.

Addington-Hall, J.M. and McCarthy, M. (1995b) Regional Study of Care for the Dying: methods and sample characteristics. *Palliat Med* 9, 27–35.

Addington-Hall, J.M., MacDonald, L.D., Anderson, H.R. and Freeling, P. (1991) Dying from cancer: the views of bereaved family and friends about the experiences of terminally ill patients. *Palliat Med* 5, 207–14.

Addington-Hall, J.M., MacDonald, L.D., Anderson, H.R., Chamberlain, J., Freeling, P., Bland, J.M., and Raftery, J. (1992) Randomised controlled trial of effects of coordinating care for terminally ill cancer patients. *BMJ* 305, 1317–22.

Addington-Hall, J.M., Weir, M.W., Zollman, C., and McIllmurray, M.B. (1993) A national survey of the provision of support services for people with cancer. *BMJ* 306, 1649–50.

Addington-Hall, J.M., Lay, M., Altmann, D. and McCarthy, M. (1995) Symptom control, communication with health professionals, and hospital care of stroke patients in the last year of life as reported by surviving family, friends, and officials. *Stroke* 26, 2242–8.

Addington-Hall, J.M., Altmann, D. and McCarthy, M. (1998a) Which terminally ill cancer patients receive hospice inpatient care? *Soc Sci Med*, 46. 1011–16.

Addington-Hall, J.M., Lay, M., Altmann, D. and McCarthy, M. (1998b) Community care for stroke patients in the last year of life: results of a national retrospective survey of surviving family, friends and officials. *Health and Social Care in the Community* 6, 112–19.

Adler, M.W. (1987) Care for patients with HIV infection and AIDS. *BMJ* 295, 27–30.

Ahmedzai, S. (1982) Dying in hospital: The residents' viewpoint. *BMJ* 285, 712–14.

Ahmedzai, S. (1990) Measuring quality of life in hospice care. *Oncology Huntingt* 4, 115–19.

Aiken, L.H. (1986) Evaluation research and public policy: lessons from the National Hospice Study. *J Chron Dis* 39, 1–4.

Albrecht, E. (1990) Palliative care in West Germany. *Palliat Med* 4, 321–5.

Aldridge, D. (1987) Families, cancer and dying. *Fam Pract* 4, 212–18.

Altman, D.G. (1991) *Practical statistics for medical research*. Chapman and Hall, London.

Amado, A.J., Grow, V., and Nofziger, J. (1995) An evaluation of hospice care with terminally ill cancer patients. *Caring* 14, 27–30.

Amenta, M.O. (1985) Hospice in the US—multiple models and varied programs. *Nurs Clin North Am* 20, 269–79.

Amesbury, B. (1990) Terminal cancer care and patients' preference for place of death. *BMJ* 301, 610–11.

Amesbury, B.D.W. (1990) Terminal care at home. *Br J Gen Pract* 40, 433.

Anand, J.K., Pryor, G.A., and Morgan, R.T.T. (1989) Hospital at home. *Health Trends* 21, 46–8.

Andrews, P.A. (1995) Palliative care for patients with terminal renal failure. *Lancet* 346, 506–7.

Anonymous (1980) National terminal care policy: Report of the working group on terminal care. *J R Coll Gen Pract* 30, 466–71.

Anonymous (1982) Study of hospice care shows need for more cost-effective services. *Hospitals* 56(9), 48.

Anonymous (1983) Les soins hospitaliers du malade en fin de vie. Etude comparative d'institutions suisses et etrangeres. [Hospital care for terminal patients. Comparative study of Swiss and foreign institutions] *Rev Med Suisse Romande* 103(2), 147–61.

Anonymous (1984a) *Patients dying in hospital*. Circular DA (84) 17. London: DHSS.

Anonymous (1984b) FNS and the hospice movement. Part two. Caring when curing fails. 'Hospice without Walls'—a practical approach. *Front Nurs Serv Q Bull* 59, 4–17.

Anonymous (1988a) The expert working group on integrated palliative care for persons with AIDS. Caring together: summary of a report submitted to Health and Welfare Canada (December 1987). *J Palliat Care* 4, 76–86.

Anonymous (1988b) *The operation and management of Macmillan nursing services*. London: Cancer Macmillan Relief Fund.

Anonymous (1989) Two more voluntary organisations for people with AIDS: Frontiers and the Black Communities AIDS Team. In Bould, M. and Peacock, G. (eds) *AIDS models of care*. London: King's Fund.

Anonymous (1990) Cancer pain relief and palliative care. Report of a WHO Expert Committee. *WHO–Tech Rep Series* **804**, 1–75.

Anonymous (1991a) [Terminal patients: their epidemiology and the problems of care noted by nurses in Calabrian hospitals. The Cantazaro Nurses' Cultural Association and the Ospedale di Matera working group]. *Riv Inferm* **10**, 223–31.

Anonymous (1991b) *South West Thames regional health authority: A framework for care of the terminally ill*. London: South West Thames Regional Health Authority.

Anonymous (1996a) Good care of the dying patient. American Medical Association Council on Scientific Affairs. *JAMA* **275**, 474–8.

Anonymous (1996b) *A structure for cancer nursing services*. London: Royal College of Nursing.

Anonymous (1997) *1995 Mortality Statistics: cause*. Series DH2 No.22. England and Wales. London: Office for National Statistics.

Aristides, M. and Shiell, A. (1993) The effects on hospital use and costs of a domiciliary palliative care nursing service. *Aust Health Rev* **16**, 405–13.

Asberg, K.H. (1980) Att do pa sjukhus—en jamforelse mellan storstadss-jukhus och landsortslasarett. [To die in a hospital-a comparison between large city hospital and country hospital] *Lakartidningen* **77**, 2191–5.

Athlin, E., Furaker, C., Jansson, L., and Norberg, A. (1993) Application of primary nursing within a team setting in the hospice care of cancer patients. *Cancer Nurs* **16**, 388–97.

Baack, C.M. (1993) Nursing's role in the nutritional care of the terminally ill: weathering the storm. *Hosp J* **9**, 1–13.

Bailes, J.S. (1995) Cost aspects of palliative cancer care. *Semin Oncol* **22**, 64–6.

Baker, M. (1992) Cost-effective management of the hospital-based hospice program. *J Nurs Admin* **22**, 40–5.

Baker, N.T. and Seager, R.D. (1991) A comparison of the psychosocial needs of hospice patients with AIDS and those with other diagnoses. *Hosp J* **7**, 61–9.

Bakke, K. and Pomietto, M. (1986) Family care when a child has late stage cancer: a research review. *Oncol Nurs Forum* **13**, 71–6.

Balfour, H.M. (1995) When does palliative care begin? A needs assessment of cancer patients with recurrent disease. *J Palliat Care* **11**, 53.

Barbarin, O.A. and Chesler, M.A. (1984) Relationships with the medical staff and aspects of satisfaction with care expressed by parents of children with cancer. *J Comm Health* **9**, 302–13.

Barrau, A. (1988) Le cout approche des sejours 'terminaux' dans les services de l'assistance publique. [The costs of terminal care in France] *Gestions Hospitalieres* **274**, 161–6.

Barrelet, L. and Jousson A.M.C. (1993) Organization of palliative care in a general hospital. *Palliat Med* **7**, 39–43.

Barzelai, L.P. (1981) Evaluation of a home based hospice. *J Fam Pract* **12**, 241–5.

Bass, D.M., Pestello, F.P., and Garland, T.N. (1984) Experiences with home hospice care: Determinants of place of death. *Death Educ* **8**, 199–222.

Bates, T., Hoy, A.M., Clark, O.G., and Laird, P.P. (1981) The St Thomas Hospital terminal support team. *Lancet* **1**, 1201–3.

Bath, G. (1989a) Planning hospital services. In Bould, M. and Peacock, G. (eds) *AIDS models of care*. London: King's Fund.

Bath, G. (1989b). Planning for AIDS in Lothian. In Bould, M. and Peacock, G. (eds) *AIDS models of care*. London: King's Fund.

Bayer, R., Callahan, D., Fletcher, J., Hodgson, T., Jennings, B., Monsees, D., Sieverts, S., and Veatch, R. (1983) The care of the terminally ill: morality and economics. *N Engl J Med* **309**, 1490–4.

Beattie, J.M. (1995) Palliative care in terminal cardiac failure: Small numbers of patients with terminal cardiac failure may make considerable demands on services. *BMJ* **310**, 1411.

Beck Friis, B. and Strang, P. (1993a) The organization of hospital-based home care for terminally ill cancer patients: the Motala model. *Palliat Med* **7**, 93–100.

Beck Friis, B. and Strang, P. (1993b) The family in hospital-based home care with special reference to terminally ill cancer patients. *J Palliat Care* **9**, 5–13.

Begg, C.B., Zelen, M., Carbone, P.P., McFadden, E.T., Brodovsky, H., Engstrom, P., Hatfield, A., Ingle, J., Schwartz, B., and Stolbach, L. (1983) Cooperative groups and community hospitals. Measurement of impact in the community hospitals. *Cancer* **52**, 1760–7.

Belonleneutre, M., Schraub, S., Mercier, M., Bourgeois, P. and Breton, C. (1988) Evaluation of health-care expenditure during 6 months after cancer—diagnosis from population registry data. *Rev Eipdemiol Sante Publique* **4–5**, 318–24.

Benjamin, A.E. (1988) Long-term care and AIDS: perspectives from experience with the elderly. *Milbank Q* **66**, 415–43.

Benjamin, A.E. and Preston, S.D. (1993) A comparative perspective on hospice care for persons with AIDS. *AIDS Public Policy J* **8**, 36–43.

Bennett, M. and Corcoran, G. (1994) The impact on community palliative care services of a hospital palliative care team. *Palliat Med* **8**, 237–44.

Bennett, P. (1984) The dying child. A care team for terminally ill children. *Nurs Times* **80**, 26–7.

Bennett, R.G. (1983) Care of the demented: long-term care institution, home and family care, and hospice. *Adv Neurol* **38**, 253–63.

Beresford, L. (1989) Alternative, outpatient settings of care for people with AIDS. *QRB Qual Rev Bull* **15**, 9–16.

Bergen, A. (1991) Nurses caring for the terminally ill in the community: a review of the literature. *Int J Nurs Stud* **28**, 89–101.

Bergen, A. (1992) Evaluating nursing care of the terminally ill in the community: a case study approach. *Int J Nurs Stud* **29**, 81–94.

Berry, D.E., Boughton, L. and McNamee, F. (1994) Patient and physician characteristics affecting the choice of home based hospice, acute care inpatient hospice facility, or hospitals as last site of care for patients with cancer of the lung. *Hosp J* **9**, 21–38.

Biedermann Hefner, M. (1991) Home care of terminal AIDS patients. *Fortschr Med* **109**, 26.

Birenbaum, L.K. and Clarke Steffen, L. (1992) Terminal care costs in childhood cancer. *Pediatr Nurs* **18**, 285–8.

Birnbaum, H.G. and Kidder, D. (1984) What does hospice care cost? *J Pub Health* **74**, 689–97.

Blaxter, M. (1995) *Consumers and research in the NHS: Consumer issues within the NHS.* Leeds: Department of Health.

Blesch, K.S. (1996) Rehabilitation of the cancer patient at home. *Semin Oncol Nurs* **12**, 219–25.

Bloom, B.S. (1987) Is hospice care least expensive for the terminally ill? *Hosp J* **3**, 67–76.

Bloom, B.S. and Kissick, P.D. (1980) Home and hospital cost of terminal illness. *Med Care* **18**, 560–4.

Bly, J.L. and Kissick, P. (1994) Hospice care for patients living alone: results of a demonstration program. *Hosp J* **9**, 9–20.

Blyth, A.C. (1990) Audit of terminal care in a general practice. *BMJ* **300**, 983–6.

Bodine, G.E. and Sobotor, W. (1980) The hospice: an integrated bibliography. *J Health Human Resources Admin* **3**, 29–55.

Boldy, D. (1989) Economic appraisal in health care with particular reference to hospice and palliative care. *Aust Health Rev* **12**, 72–6.

Bonham, G.S., Gochman, D.S., and Burgess, L. (1987) Hospice in transition: Kentucky 1982–85. *Am J Public Health* **77**, 1535–6.

Boomla, D. (1987) *Care of the dying: a guide for Health Authorities.* King's Fund/NAHA working party. London: NAHA.

Bould, M. and Peacock, G. (1989) *AIDS models of care*. King's Fund, London Boroughs Training Committee, Terrence Higgins Trust and Frontliners. London: King's Fund.

Boyd, K. (1992) The working patterns of hospice based home care teams. *Palliat Med* **6**, 131–9.

Boyd, K.J. (1993) Short terminal admissions to a hospice. *Palliat Med* **7**, 289–94.

Boyd, K.J. (1994) Hospice home care in the United Kingdom. *Ann Acad Med Singapore* **23**, 271–4.

Boyd, K.J. (1995) The role of specialist home care teams: views of general practitioners in south London. *Palliat Med* **9**, 138–44.

Boyle, D.M. (1994a) New identities: the changing profile of patients with cancer, their families, and their professional caregivers. *Oncol Nurs Forum* **21**, 55–61.

Boyle, D.M. (1994b) Realities to guide novel and necessary nursing care in geriatric oncology. *Cancer Nurs* **17**, 125–36.

Boyle, D.M. (1995) Documentation and outcomes of advanced nursing practice. *Oncol Nurs Forum* **22**, 11–17.

Braby, T. (1995) Palliative care in motor neurone disease. *Int J Pall Nurs* **1**, 183–8.

Bradshaw, P.J. (1993) Characteristics of clients referred to home, hospice and hospital palliative care services in Western Australia. *Palliat Med* **7**, 101–7.

Bramwell, L., MacKenzie, J., Laschinger, H., and Cameron, N. (1995) Need for overnight respite for primary caregivers of hospice clients. *Cancer Nurs* **18**, 337–43.

Brazil, K. and Thomas, D. (1995) The role of volunteers in a hospital-based palliative care service. *J Palliat Care* **11**, 40–2.

Brechling, B.G. and Kuhn, D. (1989) A specialised hospice for dementia patients and their families. *J Hosp Care* **6**, 27–30.

Brege, J.A. (1985a) Terminal care: A bibliography of the psychosocial literature. *Hosp J* **1**(3), 51–79.

Brege, J.A. (1985b) Terminal care: A bibliography of the medical and nursing literature. *Hosp J* **1**(4), 55–76.

Breindel, C.L. and Acree, C.L. (1980) Estimates of need for hospice services. *Death Educ* **4**, 215–22.

Brescia, F., Sadof, M. and Barstow, J. (1984) Retrospective analysis of a home care hospice program. *Omega: J of death and dying* **15**, 37–44.

Briggs, J.S. (1987) Volunteer qualities: a survey of hospice volunteers. *Oncol Nurs Forum* **14**, 27–31.

Broadfield, L. (1988) Evaluation of palliative care: current status and future directions. *J Palliat Care* **4**, 21–8.

Bromberg, M.H. and Higginson, I.J. (1996) Bereavement follow-up: What do palliative support teams actually do? *J Palliat Care* **12**, 12–17.

Brooks, C.H. (1983) The potential cost savings of hospice care: a review of the literature. *Health Matrix* **1**, 49–53.

Brooks, C.H. (1989) Cost differences between hospice and nonhospice care. A comparison of insurer payments and provider charges. *Eval Health Prof* **12**, 159–78.

Brooks, C.H. and SmythStaruch, K. (1984) Hospice home care cost savings to third-party insurers. *Med Care* **22**, 691–703.

Brown, P., Davies, B., and Martens, N. (1990) Families in supportive care—Part II: Palliative care at home: a viable care setting. *J Palliat Care* **6**, 21–7.

Bruera, E. (1989) Influence of the pain and symptom control team on the patterns of treatment of pain and other symptoms in a cancer centre. *J Pain Symptom Manage* **4**, 112–16.

Bruera, E., Kuehn, N., Emery, B., Macmillan, K., and Hanson, J. (1990a) Social and demographic characteristics of patients admitted to a palliative care unit. *J Palliat Care* **6**, 16–20.

Bruera, E., Macmillan, K., Hanson, J., and MacDonald, R.N. (1990b) Palliative care in a cancer center: Results in 1984 versus 1987. *J Pain Symptom Manage* **5**, 1–5.

Bruera, E., Kuehn, N., Selmser, P., and Macmillan, K. (1991) The Edmonton symptom assessment system (ESAS) a simple method for the assessment of palliative care patients. *J Palliat Care* **7**, 6–9.

Bruster, S., Jarman, B., Bosanquet, N., Weston, D., Erens, R. and Delbanco, T.I. (1994) National survey of hospital patients. *BMJ* **309**, 1542–9.

Buckingham, R.W. and Lupu, D. (1982) A comparative study of hospice services in the United States. *Am J Public Health* **72**, 455–63.

Bulkin, W., Brown, L., Fraioli, D., Giannattasio, E., McGuire, G., Tyler, P., and Friedland, G. (1988) Hospice care of the intravenous drug user AIDS patient in a skilled nurse facility. *J Acquir Immune Defic Syndr* **1**, 375–80.

Bullinger, M. (1992) Quality of life assessment in palliative care. *J Palliat Care* **8**, 34–9.

Burman, M.E., Steffes, M., and Weinert, C. (1993) Cancer home care in Montana. *Home Health Care Serv Q* **14**, 37–52.

Burnard, P. (1993) The psychosocial needs of people with HIV and AIDS: a view from nurse educators and counsellors. *J Adv Nurs* **18**, 1779–86.

Burne, S.R. (1984) A hospice for children in England. *Pediatrics* **73**, 97–8.

Butters, E., Higginson, I., and George, R. (1991) Two community HIV/ AIDS teams: referrals, patient characteristics and pattern of care. *Health Trends* **23**, 59–62.

Butters, E., Higginson, I., George, R., Smits, A., and McCarthy, M. (1992) Assessing the symptoms, anxiety and practical needs of HIV/AIDS patients receiving palliative care. *Qual Life Res* **1**, 47–51.

Butters, E., Higginson, I., George, R., and McCarthy, M. (1993) Palliative care for people with HIV/AIDS: views of patients, carers and providers. *AIDS Care* **5**, 105–16.

Byock, I.R. (1984) Hospice and the family physician. *J Fam Pract* **18**, 781–4.

Byrd, S. and Taylor, K. (1989) Evaluating a hospice program: a practical approach. *Am J Hosp Care* **6**, 41–6.

Byrne, C.M. (1984) Needs assessment and hospice planning in a rural setting. *Eval Health Prof* **7**, 205–19.

Caldwell, J. and Scott, J.P. (1994) Effective hospice volunteers: demographic and personality characteristics. *Am J Hosp Palliat Care* **11**, 40–5.

Calman, F.M.B. and Dobbs, H.J. (1994) Access to specialist palliative care. Purchasers come between complementary specialties. *BMJ* **308**, 656.

Campbell, M.L. (1996) Program assessment through outcomes analysis: efficacy of a comprehensive supportive care team for end-of-life care. *AACN Clin Issues* **7**, 159–67.

Campbell, M.L. and Field, B.E. (1991) Management of the patient with do not resuscitate status: Compassion and cost containment. *Heart Lung: J Crit Care* **20**, 345–8.

Carbone, P.P. (1985) Organization of clinical oncology in the U.S.A.: role of cancer centers, cooperative groups and community hospitals. *Eur J Cancer Clin Oncol* **21**, 149–54.

Carlson, R.W., Devich, L., and Frank, R.R. (1988) Development of a comprehensive supportive care team for the hopelessly ill on a university hospital medical service. *JAMA* **259**, 378–83.

Carney, K. (1981) An economic perspective on hospices. *Socioecon Issues Health* 93–108.

Carney, K. and Burns, N. (1991) Economics of hospice care. *Oncol Nurs Forum* **18**, 761–8.

Carney, K., Brobst, B., and Burns, N. (1989) The impact of reimbursement: the case of hospice. *Hosp J* **5**, 73–91.

Cartwright, A. (1990) *The role of the general practitioner in caring for people in the last year of their lives.* London: King's Fund.

Cartwright, A. (1991a) Changes in life and care in the year before death 1969–1987. *J Public Health Med* **13**, 81–7.

Cartwright, A. (1991b) The relationship between GP's hospital consultants and community nurses when caring for people in the last year of their lives. *Fam Pract* **8**, 350–5.

Cartwright, A. (1991c) The role of residential nursing homes in the last year of people's lives. *Br J Soc Work* **21**, 627–45.

Cartwright, A. (1992a) Social class differences in health and care in the year before death. *J Epidemiology Comm Health* **46**, 54–7.

Cartwright, A. (1992b) Changes in the year before death 1969–87. *Nurs Times* **88**, 51.

Cartwright, A. (1993) Dying when you're old. *Age Ageing* **22**, 425–30.

Cartwright, A. and Seale, C.F. (1990) *The natural history of a survey: an account of the methodological issues encountered in a study of life before death.* London: King's Fund.

Cella, D.F. (1995) Measuring quality of life in palliative care. *Semin Oncol* **22**, 73–81.

Chambers, E.J. and Oakhill, A. (1995) Models of care for children dying of malignant disease. *Palliat Med* **9**, 181–5.

Chambers, E.J., Oakhill, A., Cornish, J.M., and Curnick, S. (1989) Terminal care at home for children with cancer. *BMJ* **298**, 937–40.

Chambers, T.L. (1987) Hospices for children? *BMJ* **294**, 1309–10.

Chan, A. and Woodruff, R.K. (1991) Palliative care in a general teaching hospital. 1. Assessment of needs. *Med J Aust* **155**, 597–9.

Cherny, N.I., Coyle, N., and Foley, K.M. (1996) Guidelines in the care of the dying cancer patient. *Hematol Oncol Clin North Am* **10**, 261–86.

Chinner, T.L. and Dalziel, F.R. (1991) An exploratory study on the viability and efficacy of a pet-facilitated therapy project within a hospice. *J Palliat Care* **7**, 13–20.

Christakis, N.A. (1994) Timing of referral of terminally ill patients to an outpatient hospice. *J Gen Intern Med* **9**, 314–20.

Clark, A. and Fallowfield, L.J. (1986) Quality of life measurements in patients with malignant disease. *J R Soc Med* **79**, 165–9.

Clark, C., Curley, A., Hughes, A., and James, R. (1988) Hospice care: a model for caring for the person with AIDS. *Nurs Clin North Am* **23**, 851–62.

Clark, D. (1994) Recent developments in palliative care policy and practice. *Physiotherapy* **80**, 854–5.

Clark, D., Neale, B., and Heather, P. (1995a) Contracting for palliative care. *Soc Sci Med* **40**, 1193–202.

Clark, D., Small, N., and Malson, H. (1995b) Palliative care. Hospices to fortune. *Health Serv J* **105**, 30–1.

Clark, D., Small, N., and Malson, H. (1996) The NHS reforms and the hospice movement: an aggregated case study of twelve UK hospices. *Palliat Med* **10**, 62.

Clench, P. (1984) *Managing to care in the community: Services for the terminally ill*, London: Patten press.

Clench, P. (1986) The development of home care services in the UK. In Spilling, R. (Ed.) *Terminal care at home*, Oxford: Oxford University Press.

Cody, C.P. and Naierman, N. (1990) Evaluation of the cost effectiveness of a collaborative liaison program. *Hosp J* 6, 47–61.

Cohen, G., Forbes, J., and Garraway, M. (1996) Can different patient satisfaction survey methods yield consistent results? Comparison of three surveys. *BMJ* 313, 841–4.

Cohen, L.M., McCue, H.D., Germain, M., and Kjellstrand, C.M. (1995) Dialysis discontinuation: a 'good death'? *Arch Intern med* 155, 42–7.

Cohen, M.Z. (1995) The meaning of cancer and oncology nursing: link to effective care. *Semin Oncol Nurs* 11, 59–67.

Cohen, M.Z., Haberman, M.R., Steeves, R., and Deatrick, J.A. (1994) Rewards and difficulties of oncology nursing. *Oncol Nurs Forum* 21, 9–17.

Cohen, S.R. and Mount, B.M. (1992) Quality of life in terminal illness: defining and measuring subjective well-being in the dying. *J Palliat Care* 8, 40–5.

Cohen, S.R., Mount, B.M., Tomas, J.J.N. and Mount, L.F. (1996) Existential well-being is an important determinant of quality of life: Evidence from the McGill Quality of Life Questionnaire. *Cancer* 77, 576–86.

Cohen, S.R., Mount, B.M., Bruera, E., Provost, M., Rowe, J., and Tong, K. (1997) Validity of the McGill Quality of Life Questionnaire in the palliative care setting: A multi-centre Canadian study demonstrating the importance of the existential domain. *Palliat Med* 11, 3–20.

Cole, R.M. (1991) Medical aspects of care for the person with advances aquired immune deficiency syndrome (AIDS): a palliative care perspective. *Palliat Med* 5, 96–111.

Collins, C. and Ogle, K. (1994) Patterns of predeath service use by dementia patients with a family caregiver. *J Am Geriatr Soc* 42, 719–22.

Collins, C.M. (1981) The Methodist Hospice program. *J Fla Med Assoc* 68, 293–8.

Connor, S.R. and Kraymer, L.K. (1982) The evolution of an urban-based hospice program. *Fam Community Health* 5 39–53.

Connors, A.F.J., Dawson, N.V., Desbiens, N.A., Fulkerson, W.J.J., Goldman, L., Knaus, W.A. *et al.* (1995) A controlled trial to improve care for seriously ill hospitalized patients: The study to understand prognoses and preferences for outcomes and risks of treatments (SUPPORT). *JAMA* 274, 1591–8.

Copp, G. and Dunn, V. (1993) Frequent and difficult problems perceived by nurses caring for the dying in community, hospice and acute care settings. *Palliat Med* 7, 19–25.

Copperman, H. (1988) Domiciliary hospice care: a survey of general practitioners. *J R Coll Gen Pract* 38, 411–13.

Corner, J. (1996) Is there a research paradigm for palliative care? *Palliat Med* 10, 201–8.

Costantini, M., Camoirano, E., Madeddu, L., Bruzzi, P., Verganelli, E., and Henriquet, F. (1993) Palliative home care and place of death among cancer patients: A population-based study. *Palliat Med* 7, 323–31.

Courtens, A.M., Stevens, F.C.J., Crevolder, H.F.J.M., and Philipsen, H. (1996) Longitudinal study on quality of life and social support in cancer patients. *Cancer Nurs* 19, 162–9.

Couvreur, C. (1988) Les soins palliatifs pour les patients au stade terminal d'un cancer. [Palliative care for terminal cancer patients] *Bulletin d'Education du Patient a sa Maladie* 7, 88–9.

Cowley, S. (1990) *To the end of their days. Care of the dying in East-bourne's Health District.* Eastbourne: Eastbourne Health Authority.

Cowley, S. (1993) Supporting dying people. *Nurs Times* 89, 52–5.

Cox, K., Bergen, A., and Norman, I.J. (1993) Exploring consumer views of care provided by the Macmillan nurse using the critical incident technique. *J Adv Nurs* 18, 408–15.

Coyle, N., Adelhardt, J., Foley, K.M., and Portenoy, R.K. (1990) Character of terminal illness in the advanced cancer patient: Pain and other symptoms during the last four weeks of life. *J Pain Symptom Manage* 5, 83–93.

Cranfield, S. (1989) Responding to the needs of drug users with AIDS. In Bould, M. and Peacock, G. (eds) *AIDS models of care.* London: King's Fund.

Creek, L.V. (1982) A homecare hospice profile: description, evaluation, and cost analysis. *J Fam Pract* 14, 53–8.

Crowther, T., Biswas, B., Randall, F., Macpherson, D., and Wells, F. (1995) *Guidelines on research in palliative care.* London: National Council for Hospice and Specialist Palliative Care Services.

Cunningham, D. (1989) Key issues for planning. In Bould, M. and Peacock, G. (eds) *AIDS models of care.* London: King's Fund.

Curtin, L.L. (1996) First you suffer, then you die: findings of a major study on dying in U.S. hospitals. *Nurs Manage* 27, 56–60.

Curtis, A.E. and Fernsler, J.I. (1989) Quality of life of oncology hospice patients: a comparison of patient and primary caregiver reports. *Oncol Nurs Forum* 16, 49–53.

Cushen, M. (1994) Palliative care in severe heart failure. *BMJ* 308, 717.

Cutcliffe, J.R. (1995) How do nurses inspire and instil hope in terminally ill HIV patients? *J Adv Nurs* 22, 888–95.

Daeffler, R.J. (1985) A framework for hospice nursing. *Hosp J* 1, 91–111.

Dand, P., Field, D., Ahmedzai, S., and Biswas, B. (1991) *Client satisfaction with care at the Leicestershire Hospice.* Paper no.2, pp. 1–31. Sheffield: Trent Palliative Care Centre.

Dauber, L.G., Margolies, E., Spangenberg, S.E. *et al.* (1980) Hospice in hospital. Interdisciplinary group for delivery of care to terminally ill in acute-care (community) hospital. *NY State J Med* 80, 1721–3.

Davidson, P., Evans, H.R., Gray, A.J. *et al.* (1981) The development of a hospice for the continuing care of cancer patients. *N Z Med J* 94, 52–4.

Davies, B. (1996) Assessment of need for a children's hospice program. *Death Stud* 20, 247–68.

Davies, B. and Eng, B. (1993) Factors influencing nursing care of children who are terminally ill: a selective review. *Pediatr Nurs* 19, 9–14.

Davies, B. and Oberle, K. (1990) Dimensions of the supportive role of the nurse in palliative care. *Oncol Nurs Forum* 17, 87–94.

Dawson, N.J. (1991) Need satisfaction in terminal care settings. *Soc Sci Med* 32, 83–7.

de Haes, H.J. and van Knippenberg, F.C.E. (1985) The quality of life of cancer patients and review of the literature. *Soc Sci Med* 20, 809–17.

Deatrick, J.A. and Fischer, D.K. (1994) The atypical becomes typical: the work of oncology nurses. *Oncol Nurs Forum* 21, 35–40.

Degner, L.F., Henteleff, P.D., and Ringer, C. (1987) The relationship between theory and measurement in evaluations of palliative care services. *J Palliat Care* 3, 8–13.

Degner, L.F., Gow, C.M., and Thompson, L.A. (1991) Critical nursing behaviors in care for the dying. *Cancer Nurs* 14, 246–53.

DeHovitz, J.A. and Pellegrino, V. (1987) AIDS care in New York city: The comprehensive care alternative. *NY State J Med* 87, 298–300.

Delbanco, T.I. (1996) Quality of care through the patient's eyes. *BMJ* 313, 832–3.

Delight, E. and Goodall, J. (1988) Babies with spina bifida treated without surgery: parents' views on home versus hospital care. *BMJ* 297, 1230–3.

Delvaux, N., Razavi, D., and Farvaques, C. (1988) Cancer care: A stress for health professionals. *Soc Sci Med* 27, 159–66.

Dessloch, A., Maiworm, M., Florin, I., and Schulze, C. (1992) Krankenhauspflege versus Hauskrankenpflege: Zur Lebensqualitat bei terminalen Tumorpatienten. [Hospital care versus home nursing: on the quality of life of terminal tumor patients] *Psychother Psychosom Med Psychol* 42, 424–9.

Devine, E.C. and Westlake, S.K. (1995) The effects of psychoeducational care provided to adults with cancer: meta-analysis of 116 studies. *Oncol Nurs Forum* 22, 1369–81.

Dicks, B. (1990) The contribution of nursing to palliative care. *Palliat Med* 4, 197–203.

Didich, J. and Weick, J.K. (1989) The development of a palliative care program. *Cleve Clin J Med* 56, 762–4.

Dobratz, M.C. (1990) Hospice nursing: Present perspectives and future directives. *Cancer Nurs* 13, 116–22.

Dobratz, M.C., Wade, R., Herbst, L., and Ryndes, T. (1991) Pain efficacy in home hospice patients. A longitudinal study. *Cancer Nurs* 14, 20–6.

Dominica, F. (1987) The role of the hospice for the dying child. *Br J Hosp Med* 38, 334–6, 340–3.

Downe-Wamboldt, B. and Ellerton, M. (1985) A study of the role of hospice volunteers. *Hosp J* 1, 17–31.

Doyle, D. (1980) Domiciliary terminal care. *Practitioner* 224, 575–82.

Doyle, D. (1982) Domiciliary terminal care: demands on statutory services. *J R Coll Gen Pract* 32, 285–91.

Doyle, D. (1991) A home care service for terminally ill patients in Edinburgh. *Health Bull Edinb* 49, 14–23.

Doyle, D, Hanks, G.W.C., and Macdonald, N. (eds) (1993) *Oxford textbook of palliative medicine*, Oxford: Oxford University Press.

Droste, T. (1987) Alternate care: Going home to die: Developing home health care service for AIDS patients. *Hospitals* 61, 54–8.

Dubos, G., Chardon Tourne, M., and Leresteux-Olive, C. (1995) Particularites dans les soins palliatifs d'une population de cent cancereux ages hospitalises dans un service de moyen sejour. [Specificities in the palliative care of a population of 100 elderly patients presenting with neoplastic disease and hospitalized in a medium-stay department] *Rev Geriatr* 20, 273–8.

Dudgeon, D.J., Raubertas, R.F., Doerner, K., O'Connor, T., Tobin, M., and Rosenthal, S.N. (1995) When does palliative care begin? A needs assessment of cancer with recurrent disease. *J Palliat Care* 11, 5–9.

Duffy, C.M., Pollock, P., Levy, M., Budd, E., Caulfield, L., and Koren, G. (1990) Home-based palliative care for children—Part 2: The benefits of an established program. *J Palliat Care* 6, 8–14.

Dunlop, R.J., Davies, R.J., and Hockley, J.M. (1989) Preferred versus actual place of death: a hospital palliative care support team experience. *Palliat Med* 3, 197–201.

Dunphy, K. and Amesbury, B. (1990) A comparison of hospice and home care patients: patterns of referral, patient characteristics and predictors of death. *Palliat Med* 4, 105–11.

Dush, D.M. and Cassileth, B.R. (1985) Program evaluation in terminal care. *Hosp J* 1, 55–72.

Edwardson, S.R. (1983) The choice between hospital and home care for terminally ill children. *Nurs Res* 32, 29–34.

Ellershaw, J.E. (1993) Motor neurone disease—Part 1. *Palliat Care Today* 2, 25–6.

Ellershaw, J.E., Peat, S.J. and Boys, L.C. (1995) Assessing the effectiveness of a hospital palliative care team. *Palliat Med* 9, 145–52.

Emanuel, E.J. (1996) Cost savings at the end of life: What do the data show? *JAMA* **275**, 1907–14.

Emanuel, E.J. and Emanuel, L.L. (1994) The economics of dying. The illusion of cost savings at the end of life. *N Engl J Med* **330**, 540–4.

Enck, R.E. (1987) Alzheimer's disease and hospice care. *Am J Hosp Care* **4**, 19–20.

Eriscsson-Persson, B., Galvan, S. and Bexell, G. (1984) Care of senile demented patients in the final stage of the disease as experienced by their close relatives. *J Clin Exp Geront* **6**, 17–26.

Erle, H.R. (1982) Terminal care. The national scene and the individual patient. *Med Clin North Am* **66**, 1161–8.

Evans, C. and McCarthy, M. (1984) Referral and survival of patients accepted by a terminal care support team. *J Epidemiology Comm Health* **38**, 310–14.

Eve, A. and Smith, A.M. (1994) Palliative care services in Britain and Ireland—update 1991. *Palliat Med* **8**, 19–27.

Eve, A. and Smith, A.M. (1996) Survey of hospice and palliative care inpatient units in the UK and Ireland, 1993. *Palliat Med* **10**, 13–21.

Expert Advisory Group on Cancer (1995) *A policy framework for commissioning cancer services. Report to the Chief Medical Officers of England and Wales.* London: Department of Health.

Faithfull, S. (1996) How many subjects are needed in a research sample in palliative care? *Palliat Med* **10**, 259–61.

Fakhoury, W.K.H. (1994) A comparison of service and non-service determinants of carers' satisfaction with palliative care. PhD thesis, London University.

Fakhoury, W.K.H., Addington-Hall, J.M. and McCarthy, M. (1996a) A comparison by age of community and hospital services received by cancer patients in their last year of life. (Unpublished).

Fakhoury, W.K.H., McCarthy, M. and Addington-Hall, J.M. (1996b) Determinants of informal caregivers' satisfaction with services for dying cancer patients. *Soc Sci Med* **42**, 721–31.

Fakhoury, W.K.H., McCarthy, M. and Addington-Hall, J.M. (1996c) Which informal carers are most satisfied with services for dying cancer patients. *Eur J Pub Health* **6**, 181–7.

Fakhoury, W.K.H., McCarthy, M. and Addington-Hall, J.M. (1997) The effects of clinical characteristics of dying patients on informal caregivers' satisfaction with palliative care. *Palliat Med* **11**(2), 107–15.

Faulkner, A., Higginson, I., Heulwen, E., Power, M., Sykes, N. and Wilkes, E. (1993) *Hospice day care: a qualitative study.* pp. 1–26. Sheffield: Trent Palliative Care Centre.

Feingold, M.G. and Meyer, J.W. (1983) Need determination and planning methodology for the inner-city hospice. *Prog Clin Biol Res* **120**, 405–15.

Ferrell, B., Grant, M., Padilla, G., Vemuri, S., and Rhiner, M. (1991) The experience of pain and perceptions of quality of life: validation of a conceptual model. *Hosp J* 7, 9–24.

Ferris, F.D., Wodinsky, H.B., Kerr, I.G., Sone, M., Hume, S., and Coons, C. (1991) A cost-minimization study of cancer patients requiring a narcotic infusion in hospital and at home. *J Clin Epidemiol* 44, 313–27.

Field, D. (1989) Nurse's accounts of nursing the terminally ill on a coronary care unit. *Intensive Care Nurs* 5, 114–22.

Field, D. (1998) Special not different: General practitioners accounts of their care of dying people. *Soc Sci Med* 46, 111–20.

Field, D. and James, N. (1993) Where and how people die. In Clark, D. (ed.) *The Future for Palliative Care*, pp. 6–29. Milton Keynes: Open University Press.

Field, D., Dand, P., Ahmedzai, S., and Biswas, B. (1992) Care and information received by lay carers of terminally ill patients at the Leicestershire Hospice. *Palliat Med* 6, 237–45.

Field, D., Douglas, C., Jagger, C., and Dand, P. (1995) Terminal illness: views of patients and their lay carers. *Palliat Med* 9, 45–54.

Finlay, H., McCarthy, M., and Dallimore, D. (1994) Setting standards for palliative care. *J R Soc Med* 87, 179–81.

Finlay, I.G. and Dunlop, R. (1994) Quality of life assessment in palliative care. *Ann Oncol* 5, 13–18.

Fitzpatrick, R. (1991a) Surveys of patient satisfaction: II—Designing a questionnaire and conducting a survey. *BMJ* 302, 1129–32.

Fitzpatrick, R. (1991b) Surveys of patient satisfaction: I—Important general considerations. *BMJ* 302, 887–9.

Fleming, C., Scanlon, C., and Agostino, N.S. (1987) A study of the comfort needs of patients with advanced cancer. *Cancer Nurs* 10, 237–43.

Flynn, A. and Stewart, D.F. (1979) Where do cancer patients die? A review of cancer deaths in Cuyahoga County, Ohio. *J Comm Health* 5, 126–30.

Forbes, K., Davis, C., and Ford, G. (eds) (1996) Managing terminal illness. *J. R Coll Phys* 30(3), 257–9.

Ford, G. (1992) A palliative care system: the Marie Curie Model. *Am J Hosp Palliat Care* 9(3), 15–17.

Ford, G. (1995) *Information for purchasers: background to available specialist palliative care services.* Occasional Paper, London: National Council for Hospice and Specialist Palliative Care Services.

Forster, L.E. and Lynn, J. (1988) Predicting life span for applicants to inpatient hospice. *Arch Intern med* 148, 2540–3.

Fortuny, I.E., Hansen, N., Dwyer, P., Fischstrom, S., Mata, J., and O'Brien, A. (1983) Hospice Care Program Metropolitan Medical Center. *Minn Med* 66, 577–9.

Foster, L.W. (1987) Hospice care: art and science evaluating primary caregiver perceptions. *Hosp J* 3, 31–45.

Fothergill Bourbonnais, F. (1988) Terminal care: A Canadian perspective. In Wilson-Barnett, J. and Raiman, J. (eds) *Nursing issues and research in terminal care*, pp. 19–33. New York: Wiley.

Fothergill Bourbonnais, F. and Wilson Barnett, J. (1992) A comparative study of intensive therapy unit and hospice nurses' knowledge on pain management. *J Adv Nurs* 17, 362–72.

Fowler, J. (1994) A welcome focus on a key relationship. Using Peplau's model in palliative care. *Prof Nurse* 10, 194–7.

Fowlie, M. and Berkeley, J. (1987) Quality of life—a review of the literature. *Fam Pract* 4, 226–34.

Foxall, M.J., Zimmerman, L., Standley, R., and Bene, B. (1990) A comparison of frequency and sources of nursing job stress perceived by intensive care, hospice and medical-surgical nurses. *J Adv Nurs* 15, 577–84.

Frankel, S. and Kammerling, M. (1990) Assessing the need for hospice beds. *Health Trends* 22, 83–6.

Fraser, I. (1985) Medicare reimbursement for hospice care: ethical and policy implications of cost-containment strategies. *J Health Politics Policy Law* 10, 565–78.

Galasko, C. (1997) Orthopaedic principles and management. In Doyle, D., Hanks, G.W.C., and Macdonald, N. (eds). *Oxford textbook of palliative medicine*. Oxford: Oxford University Press.

Gallup, D.G., Labudovich, M., and Zambito, P.R. (1982) The gynecologist and the dying cancer patient. *Am J Obstet Gynecol* 144, 154–61.

Gannon, C. (1995) Palliative care in terminal cardiac failure: Hospices cannot fulfil such a vast and diverse role. *BMJ* 310, 1410–11.

Garbier Heidemann, E. (1982) Services for the dying: The planner's approach to models of care. *World Hospitals* 18, 48–51.

Gardner Nix, J.S., Brodie, R., Tjan, E., Wilton, M., Zoberman, L., Barnes, F., Friedrich, J., and Wood, J. (1995) Scarborough's Palliative 'At-home' Care Team (PACT): a model for a suburban physician palliative care team. *J Palliat Care* 11, 43–9.

Garland, T.N., Bass, D.M., and Otto, M.E. (1984) The needs of hospice patients and primary caregivers: comparison of primary caregivers' and hospice nurses' perceptions. *Am J Hosp Care* 1, 40–5.

Gates, G.R. (1982) Terminal care in country practice. *Aust Fam Phys* 11, 338–42.

Gau, D.W. and Diehl, A.K. (1982) Disagreement among general practitioners regarding cause of death. *BMJ* 284, 239–41.

George, R. (1989) The Bloomsbury Care Committee. In Bould, M. and Peacock, G. (eds) *AIDS models of care*. London: King's Fund.

George, R.J.D. and Jennings, A.L. (1993) Palliative medicine. *Postgrad Med J* **69**, 429–49.

Gibson, D.E. (1984) Hospice: morality and economics. *Gerontologist* **24**, 4–8.

Gilmore, N. (1987) AIDS palliative care: the courage to care. *J Palliat Care* **3**, 33–8.

Glare, P.A. (1994) Palliative care in acquired immunodeficiency syndrome (AIDS): problems and practicalities. *Ann Acad Med Singapore* **23**, 235–43.

Glare, P.A. and Lickiss, J.N. (1992) Quality assurance in palliative care. *Med J Aust* **157**, 572.

Glickman, E.F. and Greene, H.L., Jr. (1984) Assessment of resident performance in a hospital-based palliative care unit. *Death Educ* **8**, 99–111.

Glickman, M. (1997) *Making palliative care better: quality improvement, multi-professional audit and standards.* Occasional Paper 12. London: National Council for Hospice and Specialist Palliative Care Services.

Gochman, D.S. and Bonham, G.S. (1988) Physicians and the hospice decision: awareness, discussion, reasons and satisfaction. *Hosp J* **4**, 25–53.

Goddard, M. and Hutton, J. (1991) Economic evaluation of trends in cancer therapy. *Int J Technol Assess Health Care* **7**, 594–693.

Goddard, M.K. (1993) The importance of assessing the effectiveness of care: the case of hospices. *J Soc Policy* **22**, 1–7.

Godkin, M.A., Krant, M.J., and Doster, N.J. (1983) The impact of hospice care on families. *Int J Psychiatry Med* **13**, 153–65.

Goldberg, R.J., Mor, V., Wiemann, M., Greer, D.S., and Hiris, J. (1986) Analgesic use in terminal cancer patients: report from the National Hospice Study. *J Chron Dis* **39**, 37–45.

Goldman, A., Beardsmore, S., and Hunt, J. (1990) Palliative care for children with cancer—Home, hospital, or hospice? *Arch Dis Child* **65**, 641–3.

Goldstone, I., Kuhl, D., Johnson, A., Le, R., and McLeod, A. (1995) Patterns of care in advanced HIV disease in a tertiary treatment centre. *AIDS Care* **7**, S47–56.

Goldstone, I.L. (1992) Trends in hospital utilization in AIDS care 1987–1991: implications for palliative care. *J Palliat Care* **8**, 22–9.

Gomas, J.M. (1993) Palliative care at home: A reality or 'mission impossible'? *Palliat Med* **7**, 45–59.

Gomez-Baptiste, X. (1992) Palliative care in Catalonia. *Palliat Med* **6**, 321–7.

Gooding, B.A., Sloan, M., and Gagnon, L. (1993) Important nurse caring behaviors: perceptions of oncology patients and nurses. *Can J Nurs Res* **25**, 65–76.

Gotay, C.C. (1983) Models of terminal care: a review of the research literature. *Clin Inves Med* 6, 131–41.

Graham, H. and Livesley, B. (1983) Dying as a diagnosis: Difficulties of communication and management in elderly patients. *Lancet* 2, 670–2.

Graves, D. and Nash, A. (1992) A friendship that inspires hope. A study of Macmillan nurses' working patterns. *Prof Nurse* 7, 478–85.

Gray, D., MacAdam, D., and Boldy, D. (1987) A comparative cost analysis of terminal cancer care in home hospice patients and controls. *J Chron Dis* 40, 801–10.

Greer, D.S. and Mor, V. (1986) An overview of National Hospice Study findings. *J Chron Dis* 39, 5–7.

Greer, D.S., Mor, V., Sherwood, S., Morris, J.N., and Birnbaum, H. (1983) National hospice study analysis plan. *J Chron Dis* 36, 737–80.

Greer, D.S., Mor, V., Morris, J.N., Sherwood, S., Kidder, D., and Birnbaum, H. (1986) An alternative in terminal care: results of the National Hospice Study. *J Chron Dis* 39, 9–26.

Greipp, M.E. (1996) SUPPORT study results—implications for hospice care. *Am J Hosp Palliat Care* 13, 38–45.

Grobe, M.E., Ahmann, D.L., and Ilstrup, D.M. (1982) Needs assessment for advanced cancer patients and their families. *Oncol Nurs Forum* 9, 26–30.

Grobe, M.E., Ilstrup, D.M., Ahmann, D.L., Miller, J.C., Gillard, M., Haycock, H., and Jacobsen, D. (1983) Evaluation of a coordinated community approach to hospice services. *Prog Clin Biol Res* 130, 411–15.

Hadlock, D.C. (1985) The hospice: Intensive care of a different kind. *Semin Oncol* 12, 357–67.

Haines, A. and Booroff, A. (1986) Terminal care at home: perspective from general practice. *BMJ* 292, 1051–3

Hall, J.A. and Dornan, M.C. (1988) What patients like about their medical care and how often they are asked: a meta-analysis of the satisfaction literature. *Soc Sci Med* 27, 935–9.

Hancock, B.W. (1992) Quality and cost in the palliative care of cancer. *Br J Cancer* 65, 141–2.

Hannan, E.L. and O'Donnell, J.F. (1984) An evaluation of hospices in the New York State Hospice Demonstration Program. *Inquiry* 21, 338–48.

Hanrahan, P. and Luchins, D.J. (1995a) Access to hospice programs in end-stage dementia: a national survey of hospice programs. *J Am Geriatr Soc* 43, 56–9.

Hanrahan, P. and Luchins, D.J. (1995b) Feasible criteria for enrolling end-stage dementia patients in home hospice care. *Hosp J* 10, 47–54.

Hardy, J.R., Turner, R., Saunders, M., and Ahern, R. (1994) Prediction of survival in a hospital-based continuing care unit. *Eur J Cancer* 30, 284–8.

Harrison, E. (1995) Nurse caring and the new health care paradigm. *J Nurs Care Qual* 9, 14–23.

Haupt, B., Hing, E., and Strahan, G. (1994) The national home and hospice care survey: 1992 summary. *Vital Health Stat* 13 1–110.

Hays, R.D. and Arnold, S. (1986) Patient and family satisfaction with care for the terminally ill. *Hosp J* 2, 129–50.

Hellinger, F.J., Fleishman, J.A., and Hsia, D.C. (1994) AIDS treatment costs during the last months of life: evidence from the ACSUS. *Health Serv Res* 29, 569–81.

Henderson, J., Goldacre, M.J., and Griffith, M. (1990) Hospital care for the elderly in the final year of life: a population based study. *BMJ* 301, 17–19.

Hendriksen, C., Lund, E., and Stromgard, E. (1987) Use of social and health services by elderly people during the terminal 18 months of life. *Scand J Soc Med* 15, 169–74.

Henley, A. (1986) *Good practice in hospital care for dying patients.* London: King's Fund.

Herd, E.B. (1990) Terminal care in a semi-rural area. *Br J Gen Pract* 40, 248–51.

Hermans, D., Lisaerde, J., and Triau, E. (1989) Sense and non-sense of a technological health care model in terminally ill demented patients. *J Palliat Care* 5, 55–8.

Herxheimer, A., Begent, R., MacLean, D. *et al.* (1985) The short life of a terminal care support team: Experience at Charing Cross Hospital. *BMJ* 290, 1877–9.

Hesse, K.A. (1995) Terminal care of the very old: Changes in the way we die. *Arch Intern med* 155, 1513–18.

Hickey, A.M., Bury, G., O'Boyle, C.A., Bradley, F., O'Kelly, F.D., and Shannon, W. (1996) A new short form individual quality of life measure (SEIQoL-DW): application in a cohort of individuals with HIV/AIDS. *BMJ* 313, 29–33.

Hicks, F. and Corcoran, G. (1993) Should hospices offer respite admissions to patients with motor neurone disease? *Palliat Med* 7, 145–50.

Higginson, I.J. (1990) *Palliative care in Bloomsbury. Report to Bloomsbury Health Authority.* London: Bloomsbury Support Team.

Higginson, I.J. (1993a) Palliative care: a review of past changes and future trends. *J Public Health Med* 15, 3–8.

Higginson, I.J. (1993b) Quality, costs and contracts of care. In Clark, D. (ed.) *The future for palliative care: Issues of policy and practice.* Milton Keynes: Open University Press.

Higginson, I.J. (1994) Clinical audit and organizational audit in palliative care. *Cancer Surv* 21, 233–45.

Higginson, I.J. (1995a) *Outcome measures in palliative care.* London: National Council for Hospice and Specialist Palliative Care Services.

Higginson, I.J. (1995b) *Health care needs assessment: Palliative and terminal care.* Winchester: Wessex Institute of Public Health Medicine.

Higginson, I.J. and Hearn, J. (1997) A multicenter evaluation of cancer pain control by palliative care teams. *J Pain Symptom Manage* 14, 29–35.

Higginson, I.J. and McCarthy, M. (1989) Evaluation of palliative care: steps to quality assurance? *Palliat Med* 3, 267–74.

Higginson, I.J. and McCarthy, M. (1993) Validity of the support team assessment schedule: do staffs' ratings reflect those made by patients or their families? *Palliat Med* 7, 219–28.

Higginson, I.J. and McCarthy, M. (1994) A comparison of two measures of quality of life: their sensitivity and validity for patients with advanced cancer. *Palliat Med* 8, 282–90.

Higginson, I.J., Wade, A., and McCarthy, M. (1988) A comparison of four outcome measures of terminal care. In Gilmore, A. and Gilmore, S. (eds) *A safer death: multidisciplinary aspects of terminal care,* pp. 205–11. New York: Plenum.

Higginson, I.J., Wade, A., and McCarthy, M. (1990) Palliative care: views of patients and their families. *BMJ* 301, 277–81.

Higginson, I.J., Butters, E., Murphy, F., and McDonnell, M. (1992a) Computer database for palliative care. *Lancet* 340, 243.

Higginson, I.J., Wade, A.M., and McCarthy, M. (1992b) Effectiveness of two palliative support teams. *J Public Health Med* 14, 50–6.

Higginson, I.J., Priest, P., and McCarthy, M. (1994a) Are bereaved family members a valid proxy for a patient's assessment of dying? *Soc Sci Med* 38, 553–7.

Higginson, I.J., Webb, D., and Lessof, L. (1994b) Reducing hospital beds for patients with advanced cancer. *Lancet* 344, 409.

Hill, D. and Penso, D. (1995) *Opening doors: Improving access to hospice and specialist palliative care services by members of the black and ethnic minority communities.* Occasional Paper 7, London: National Council for Hospice and Specialist Palliative Care Services.

Hill, F. and Oliver, C. (1988) Hospice—an update on the cost of patient care. *Health Trends* 20, 83–7.

Hilton, T., Orr, R.D., Perkin, R.M., and Ashwal, S. (1993) End of life care in Duchenne muscular dystrophy. *Pediatr Neurol* 9, 165–77.

Hiltunen, E.F., Puopolo, A.L., Marks, G.K., Marsden, C., Kennard, M.J., Follen, M.A., and Phillips, R.S. (1995) The nurse's role in end-of-life treatment discussions: preliminary report from the SUPPORT Project. *J Cardiovasc Nurs* 9, 68–77.

Hinton, J. (1979) Comparison of places and policies for terminal care. *Lancet* 1, 29–32.

Hinton, J. (1994a) Can home care maintain an acceptable quality of life for patients with terminal cancer and their relatives? *Palliat Med* 8, 183–96.

Hinton, J. (1994b) Which patients with terminal cancer are admitted from home care? *Palliat Med* 8, 197–210.

Hinton, J. (1996) Services given and help perceived during home care for terminal cancer. *Palliat Med* 10, 125–34.

Hjelmerus, L. (1987) Care of the dying: Present situation in Sweden. *Hosp J* 3, 91–5.

Hockey, L. (1994) Saint Columba's hospice home care service: an evaluation study. *Palliat Med* 5, 315–22.

Hockley, J. (1989) Caring for the dying in acute hospitals. *Nurs Times* 85, 47–50.

Hockley, J. (1990) Palliative care teams. *Palliat Med* 4, (editorial).

Hockley, J. (1992) Role of the hospital support team. *Br J Hosp Med* 48, 250–3.

Hockley, J. (1996) The development of a palliative care team at the Western General Hospital, Edinburgh. *Support Care Cancer* 4, 77–81.

Hockley, J.M., Dunlop, R., and Davies, R.J. (1988) Survey of distressing symptoms in dying patients and their families in hospital and the response to a symptom control team. *BMJ* 296, 1715–17.

Hodgson, L.A. (1995) Nurses working 12-hour shifts in the hospice setting. *Palliat Med* 9, 153–63.

Hofman, A., Rocca, W.A., and Brayne, C. (1991) The prevalence of dementia in Europe. *Int J Epidemiol* 20, 736–48.

Hohl, D. (1994) Patient satisfaction in home care/hospice. *Nurs Manage* 25, 52–4.

Holden, T. (1980) Patiently speaking. *Nurs Times* 1035–6.

Hopwood, P. and Stephens, R.J. (1995) Symptoms at presentation for treatment in patients with lung cancer: implications for the evaluation of palliative treatment. The Medical Research Council (MRC) Lung Cancer Working Party. *Br J Cancer* 71, 633–6.

Hopwood, P., Howell, A., and Maguire, P. (1991) Psychiatric morbidity in patients with advanced cancer of the breast: prevalence measured by two self-rating questionnaires. *Br J Cancer* 64, 349–52.

Hornsey, J. (1994) Empowering patient and carer through terminal MND. *Nurs Times* 90, 37–9.

Horsley, G.C. and Brown, J.K. (1985) Strengths and needs of per diem hospice personnel. *Cancer Nurs* 8, 43–9.

Hoskin, P.J. and Hanks, G.W. (1988) The management of symptoms in advanced cancer: experience in a hospital-based continuing care unit. *J R Soc Med* 81, 341–4.

Hospice Information Service (1996) *Hospice and palliative care: A guide to the development of the hospice movement.* London: St Christopher's Hospice.

Hospice Information Service (1997a) *Directory of Hospice and Palliative Care Services,* 1997 edn. London: St.Christopher's Hospice.

Hospice Information Service (1997b) *Hospice facts and figures 1997.* London: St Christopher's Hospice.

House, N. (1993) Helping to reach an understanding. Palliative care for people from ethnic minority groups. *Prof Nurse* 8, 329–32.

Houts, P.S., Yasko, J.M., Harvey, H.A., Kahn, S.B., Hartz, A.J., Hermann, J.F., Schelzel, G.W., and Bartholomew, M.J. (1988) Unmet needs of persons with cancer in Pennsylvania during the period of terminal care. *Cancer* 62, 627–34.

Howard, G.C., Clarke, K., and Elia, M.H. (1995) A Scottish national mortality study assessing cause of death, quality of and variation in management of patients with testicular non- seminomatous germ-cell tumours. *Br J Cancer* 72, 1307–11.

Hubbard, S.M. (1995) Clinical research and cancer nursing. *Oncol Nurs Forum* 22, 505–14.

Hudson, J.E. (1990) A profile of Canadian hospital-based palliative care. *Am J Hosp Palliat Care* 7, 35–41.

Hughes, S.L., Cummings, J., Weaver, F., Manheim, L., Braun, B., and Conrad, K. (1992) A randomized trial of the cost effectiveness of VA hospital-based home care for the terminally ill. *Health Serv Res* 26, 801–17.

Hull, M.M. (1989) Family needs and supportive nursing behaviors during terminal cancer: a review. *Oncol Nurs Forum* 16, 787–92.

Hull, M.M. (1991) Hospice nurses. Caring support for caregiving families. *Cancer Nurs* 14, 63–70.

Hunt, J.A. (1995) The paediatric oncology community nurse specialist: the influence of employment location and funders on models of practice. *J Adv Nurs* 22, 126–33.

Hunt, M. (1992) The identification and provision of care for the terminally ill at home by family members. *Sociology Health and Illness* 13, 375–95.

Hunt, R. and McCaul, K. (1996) A population-based study of the coverage of cancer patients by hospice services. *Palliat Med* 10, 5–12.

Hurley, A.C., Volicer, B., Mahoney, M.A., and Volicer, L. (1993) Palliative fever management in Alzheimer patients. quality plus fiscal responsibility. *ANS Adv Nurs Sci* 16, 21–32.

Ingleton, C. and Faulkner, A. (1993) Audit issues in palliative care: the perspective of senior nurses. *J Cancer Care* 2, 201–6.

Ingleton, C. and Faulkner, A. (1995a) Quality assurance in palliative care: some of the problems. *Eur J Cancer Care* 4, 38–44.

Ingleton, C. and Faulkner, A. (1995b) Quality assurance in palliative care—a review of the literature. *J Cancer Care* **4**, 49–55.

Ingleton, C., Field, D., Carradice, M., and Crowther, T. (1996) Multi-disciplinary evaluation of one inpatient hospice unit. *Palliat Med* **10**, 67–8.

Irvine, B. (1993) Developments in palliative nursing in and out of the hospital setting. *Br J Nurs* **2**, 218–24.

Jackson, F. and Duffy, S.A. (1994) Productivity of hospice nurses. *Am J Hosp Palliat Care* **11**, 23–6.

Jakobsen, A., Bondevik, H., Sodal, G., Jervell, J., Thorsby, E., and Flatmark, A. (1982) Organization for the care of patients with terminal renal-failure in norway. *Transplant Proc* **1**, 216–17.

James, M.L., Gebski, V.J., and Gunz, F.W. (1985) The need for palliative care services in a general hospital. *Med J Aust* **142**, 448–9.

Jarvis, H., Burge, F.I., and Scott, C.A. (1996) Evaluating a palliative care program: methodology and limitations. *J Palliat Care* **12**, 23–33.

Johnson, A. (1989) The shift to community care for people with AIDS. In Bould, M. and Peacock, G. (eds) *AIDS models of care*. London: King's Fund.

Johnson, B.A. and Smith, H.L. (1981) A strategy for integrating hospice, hospital care. *Hosp Prog* **62** 52–6.

Johnson, H. and Oliver, D. (1991) The development of palliative care services place of death of cancer patients. *Palliat Med* **5**, 40–5.

Johnson, I.S., Rogers, C., Biswas, B., and Ahmedzai, S. (1990) What do hospices do? A survey of hospices in the United Kingdom and Republic of Ireland. *BMJ* **300**, 791–3.

Johnson, L.R., Cohen, M.Z., and Hull, M.M. (1994) Cultivating expertise in oncology nursing: methods, mentors, and memories. *Oncol Nurs Forum* **21**, 27–34.

Johnston, G. and Abraham, C. (1995) The WHO objectives for palliative care: to what extent are we achieving them? *Palliat Med* **9**, 123–37.

Jones, A., Faulkner, A., and Nightingale, S.A. (1994) *Who cares? Palliative care review for United Health Commission by Grimsby and Scunthorpe Health Authority*. Occasional Paper No. 15, pp. 1–100. Sheffield: Trent Palliative Care Centre.

Jones, R.V.H., Hansford, J., and Fiske, J. (1993) Death from cancer at home: the carer's perspective. *BMJ* **306**, 249–51.

Jones, S. (1995) Palliative care in terminal cardiac failure. *BMJ* **310**, 805.

Jupp, M.R. (1994) Management review of nursing systems. *J Nurs Manag* **2**, 57–64.

Kaiser, C.B. (1984) Hospice inpatient care: Characteristics of an institution and its patients. *Conn Med* **48**, 146–51.

Kane, R.L. (1986) Lessons from hospice evaluations. *Hosp J* **2**, 3–8.

Kane, R.L., Wales, J., Bernstein, L., Leibowitz, A., and Kaplan, S. (1984) A randomised controlled trial of hospice care. *Lancet* 1, 890–4.

Kane, R.L., Berstein, L., Wales, J., and Rothenberg, R. (1985a) Hospice effectiveness in controlling pain. *JAMA* 253, 2683–6.

Kane, R.L., Klein, S.J., Bernstein, L., Rothenberg, R., and Wales, J. (1985b) Hospice role in alleviating the emotional stress of terminal patients and their families. *Med Care* 23, 189–97.

Kane, R.L., Klein, S.J., Bernstein, L., and Rothenberg, R. (1986) The role of hospice in reducing the impact of bereavement. *J Chron Dis* 39, 735–42.

Kaplan, M.P. and O'Connor, P. (1989) Hospital care for minorities: an analysis of a hospital-based inner city palliative care service. *Am J Hosp Care* 6, 13–21.

Kaplan, R.M. (1993) Quality of life assessment for cost/utility studies in cancer. *Cancer Treat Rev* 19 Suppl A, 85–96.

Kaplow, R. (1996) The role of the advanced practice nurse in the care of patients critically ill with cancer. *AACN Clin Issues* 7, 120–30.

Keay, T.J., Fredman, L., Taler, G.A., Datta, S., and Levenson, S.A. (1994) Indicators of quality medical care for the terminally ill in nursing homes. *J Am Geriatr Soc* 42, 853–60.

Keith, P.M. and Castles, M.R. (1979) Expected and observed behavior of nurses and terminal patients. *Int J Nurs Stud* 16, 21–8.

Keizer, M.C., Kozak, J.F., and Scott, J.F. (1992) Primary care providers' perceptions of care. *J Palliat Care* 8, 8–12.

Kellar, N., Martinez, J., Finis, N., Bolger, A., and von Gunten, C.F. (1996) Characterization of an acute inpatient hospice palliative care unit in a U.S. teaching hospital. *J Nurs Admin* 26, 16–20.

Kelly, M. and Barber, H. (1989) Comparing urban and rural hospice services. *Practitioner* 233, 1063–5.

Kelly, M. and Cats, M. (1994) Hospice care in motor neurone disease. *Nurs Stand* 9, 30–2.

Kelson, M. (1995) *Consumer involvement initiatives in clinical audit and outcomes.* London: College of Health.

Kemp, C. and Stepp, L. (1995) Palliative care for patients with acquired immunodeficiency syndrome. *Am J Hosp Palliat Care* 12, 14, 17–27.

Kidder, D. (1992) The effects of hospice coverage on Medicare expenditures. *Health Serv Res* 27, 195–217.

Kincade, J.E. and Powers, R. (1984) An assessment of palliative care needs in a tertiary care hospital. *QRB Qual Rev Bull* 10, 230–7.

Kindlen, M. (1988) Hospice home care services: a Scottish perspective. *Palliat Med* 2, 115–21.

King, M., Lapsley, I., Llewellyn, S., Tierney, A., Anderson, J., and Sladden, S. (1993) Purchasing palliative care: availability and cost implications. *Health Bull* 51, 370–84.

Kinzbrunner, B.M. (1994) Hospice: what to do when anti-cancer therapy is no longer appropriate, effective, or desired. *Semin Oncol* **21**, 792–8

Kirkham, S. (1992) Bed occupancy, patient throughput and size of independent hospice units in the UK. *Palliat Med* **6**, 47–53.

Kleeberg, U.R., V Kerekjarto, M., Kaden, H., Wagner-Bastmeyer, R., Kur, A., Lehmann, G., Schulz, K., Bogan, G., Reichel, L., and Erdmann, H. (1991) Supportive care of the terminally ill cancer patient at home and in a day-hopice. *Onkologie* **14**, 240–6.

Koffman, J., Higginson, I., and Naysmith, A. (1996) Hospice at home—a new service for patients with advanced HIV/AIDS: a pilot evaluation of referrals and outcomes. *Br J Gen Pract* **46**, 539–40.

Kohler, J.A. and Radford, M. (1985) Terminal care for children dying of cancer: quantity and quality of life. *BMJ* **291**, 115–16.

Komesaroff, P.A., Moss, C.K., and Fox, R.M. (1989) Patients' socio-economic background: influence on selection of inpatient or domiciliary hospice terminal-care programmes. *Med J Aust* **151**, 196–201.

Koopmanschap, M.A., van Ineveld, B.M., and Miltenburg, T.E. (1992) Costs of home care for advanced breast and cervical cancer in relation to cost-effectiveness of screening. *Soc Sci Med* **35**, 979–85.

Kovacs, P.J. and Rodgers, A.Y. (1995) Meeting the social service needs of persons with AIDS: hospices' response. *Hosp J* **10**, 49–65.

Kramer, J.A. and Dwyer, B.E. (1989) Palliative care in the teaching hospital. *Aust Cancer Soc Cancer Forum* **13**, 4–21.

Kriebel, M. (1989) A profile of hospice programs in Pennsylvania. *Hosp J* **5**, 51–71.

Krishnasamy, M. (1996) What do cancer patients identify as supportive and unsupportive behaviour of nurses? A pilot study. *Eur J Cancer Care* **5**, 103–10.

Kristjanson, L.J. (1989) Quality of terminal care: salient indicators identified by families *J Palliat Care* **5**, 21–30.

Kristjanson, L.J. and Ashcroft, T. (1994) The family's cancer journey: a literature review. *Cancer Nurs* **17**, 1–17.

Kristjanson, L.J. and Balneaves, L. (1995) Directions for palliative care nursing in Canada: report of a national survey. *J Palliat Care* **11**, 5–8.

Kubler Ross, E. (1989) *On death and dying.* London: Routledge.

Kurti, L.G. and O'Dowd, T.C. (1995) Dying of non-malignant diseases in general practice. *J Palliat Care* **11**, 25–31.

Laliberte, L.L. and Mor, V. (1985) An examination of the relationship of reimbursement and organisational structure to the use of hospice volunteers. *Hosp J* **1**, 21–44.

Lamkin, L. (1993) Assessment, development, and evaluation of cancer programs. *Semin Oncol Nurs* **9**, 17–24.

Lande, R. (1989) The role of the general practitioner in the care of people with HIV infection and AIDS. In Bould, M. and Peacock, G. (eds) *AIDS models of care*. London: King's Fund.

Latimer, E. (1991) Auditing the hospital care of dying patients. *J Palliat Care* 7, 12–17.

Laudico, A.V. (1993) The Philippines: status of cancer pain and palliative care. *J Pain Symptom Manage* 8, 429–30.

Lauer, M.E. and Camitta, B.M. (1980) Home care for dying children: a nursing model. *J Pediatr* 97, 1032–5.

Lauer, M.E., Mulhern, R.K., Hoffmann, R.G., and Camitta, B.M. (1986) Utilization of hospice/home care in pediatric oncology. A national survey. *Cancer Nurs* 9, 102–7.

Lauer, M.E., Mulhern, R.K., Wallskog, J.M., and Camitta, B.M. (1983) A comparison study of parental adaptation following a child's death at home or in the hospital. *Pediatrics* 71, 107–12.

Layzell, S. and McCarthy, M. (1993) Specialist or generic community nursing care for HIV/AIDS patients? *J Adv Nurs* 18, 531–7.

Lee, G. and Bosenquet, N. (1992) *Improving quality of life for cancer patients*. Cambridge: Daniels.

Lefroy, R.B. (1992) Palliative care in a general teaching hospital. *Med J Aust* 156, 438.

Levy, M., Duffy, C.M., Pollock, P., Budd, E., Caulfield, L., and Koren, G. (1990) Home-based palliative care for children—Part 1: The institution of a program. *J Palliat Care* 6, 11–15.

Levy, M.H. (1993) Living with cancer: hospice/palliative care. *J Nat Cancer Inst* 85, 1283–7.

Lichter, I. (1990) Palliative care services in New Zealand. *Palliat Med* 4, 219–23.

Lickiss, J.N., Wiltshire, J., Glare, P.A., and Chye, R.W. (1994) Central Sydney Palliative Care Service: potential and limitations of an integrated palliative care service based in a metropolitan teaching hospital. *Ann Acad Med Singapore* 23, 264–70.

Lickiss, N., Glare, P., Turner, K., Gibson, S., Ng, M., Macaulay, P., Formby, F., and Hartley, J. (1993) Palliative care in central Sydney: the Royal Prince Alfred Hospital as catalyst and integrator. *J Palliat Care* 9, 33–42.

Lieberman, J. (1986) AIDS. Home care hospice program. *Calif Nurse* 82, 6–7.

Lipton, H.L. (1987) Medical care in the last year of life: a review of economic and ethical issues. *Compr Gerontol B* 1, 89–93.

Lithman, T., Noreen, D., Norlund, A., and Sundstrom, B. (1994) Doende far stor del av vardresurserna. Kostnadsanalys av varden i livets slutskede. [A substantial part of health resources is reserved for the dying. Cost analysis of terminal care] *Lakartidningen* **91**, 4390–2.

Lloyd-Williams, M. (1996a) An audit of palliative care in dementia. *Eur J Cancer Care* **5**, 53–5.

Lloyd-Williams, M. (1996b) A survey of palliative care given to patients with end-stage dementia (abstract). *Palliat Med* **10**, 63.

Locker, D. and Dunt, D. (1978) Theoretical and methodological issues in sociological studies of consumer satisfaction with medical care. *Soc Sci Med* **12**, 283–92.

Loomis, M.T. and Williams, T.F. (1983) Evaluation of care provided to terminally ill patients. *Gerontologist* **23**, 493–9.

Lovel, T. (1996) The delivery of palliative care. *Cancer Treat Rev* **22**, 145–9.

Lubin, S. (1992) Palliative care—could your patient have been managed at home? *J Palliat Care* **8**, 18–22.

Lubitz, J. and Prihoda, R. (1984) The use and costs of Medicare services in the last 2 years of life. *Health Care Financ Rev* **5**, 117–31.

Luchins, D.J. and Hanrahan, P. (1993) What is appropriate health care for end-stage dementia?. *J Am Geriatr Soc* **41**, 25–30.

Lukashok, H. (1990) Hospice care under Medicare—an early look. *Prev Med* **19**, 730–6.

Lunceford, J.L. (1983) *A preliminary look at hospice costs.* Bethesda, Md: DHHS.

Lundahl, S.L. (1984) Development and evaluation of a community cancer resource directory. *Public Health Rep* **99**, 590–7.

Lunt, B. (1980) Where people die. *Nursing* **34**, 1479–80.

Lunt, B. (1985) Terminal cancer care services: recent changes in regional inequalities in Great Britain. *Soc Sci Med* **20**, 753–9.

Lunt, B. and Hillier, R. (1981) Terminal care: present services and future priorities. *BMJ* **283**, 595–8.

Lunt, B. and Neale, C. (1987) A comparison of hospice and hospital care goals set by staff. *Palliat Med* **1**, 136–48.

Lunt, B. and Yardley, J. (1988) *Home care teams and hospital support teams for the terminally ill.* Southampton: Royal Hants Hospital, Cancer Care Unit.

Mabbott, A. and Rothery, H. (1988) Terminal care. *Practitioner* **232**, 459–60.

Maccabee, J. (1994) The effect of transfer from a palliative care unit to nursing homes—are patients' and relatives' needs met? *Palliat Med* **8**, 211–14.

Macdonald, E.T. and Macdonald, J.B. (1992) How do local doctors react to a hospice? *Health Bull Edinb* **50**, 351–5.

MacDonald, L.D. (1989) A new scheme for the care of terminally ill cancer patients. *MRC* **44**, 12.

MacDonald, L.D., Addington-Hall, J.M., and Anderson, H.R. (1994) Acceptability and perceived effectiveness of a district co-ordinating service for terminal care: implications for quality assurance. *J Adv Nurs* **20**, 337–43.

MacDonald, N. (1991) Cure and care: interaction between cancer centers and palliative care units. *Recent Results Cancer Res* **121**, 399–407.

Maddocks, I. (1990) Changing concepts in palliative care. *Med J Aust* **152**, 535–9.

Maddocks, I., Bentley, L., and Sheedy, J. (1994) Quality of life issues in patients dying from haematological diseases. *Ann Acad Med Singapore* **23**, 244–8.

Magno, J. (1992) USA hospice care in the 1990s. *Palliat Med* **6**, 158–65.

Maguire, P. and Selby, P. (1989) MRC cancer therapy committee working party: assessing quality of life in cancer patients. *Br J Cancer* **60**, 437–40.

Maguire-Eisen, M. and Frost, C. (1994) Knowledge of malignant melanoma and how it relates to clinical practice among nurse practitioners and dermatology and oncology nurses. *Cancer Nurs* **17**, 457–63.

Maher, E.J. (1990) The role of the palliative care unit in the organization of services to patients with cancer. *Palliat Med* **4**, 293–8.

Mahon, S.M. (1991) Managing the psychosocial consequences of cancer recurrence: implications for nurses. *Oncol Nurs Forum* **18**, 577–83.

Mahoney, J.J. (1986) Lessons from hospice evaluations: counterpoint. *Hosp J* **2**, 9–15.

Malden, L.T., Sutherland, C., Tattersall, M.H., Morgan, J., Forsyth, S., Levi, J.A., and Gunz, F.W. (1984) Dying of cancer. Factors influencing the place of death of patients. *Med J Aust* **141**, 147–50.

Maletta, G.J. (1995) Access to hospice programs in end-stage dementia. *J Am Geriatr Soc* **43**, 1174–5.

Malson, H., Clark, D., Small, N. and Mallett, K. (1996) The impact of NHS reforms on UK palliative care services. *Eur J Palliat Care* **3**, 68–71.

Manning, M. (1984) *The hospice alternative*. London: Souvenir Press.

Mansfield, S., Barter, G., and Singh, S. (1992) AIDS and palliative care. *Int J STD AIDS* **3**, 248–50.

Martens, N. and Davies, B. (1990) The work of patients and spouses in managing advanced cancer at home. *Hosp J* **6**, 55–73.

Martin, E.W. and Soja, E.W. (1989) Symptom management in the home-based terminal cancer patient. *R I Med J* **72**, 243–52.

Martin, J.P. (1986) The AIDS home care and hospice program. A multidisciplinary approach to caring for persons with AIDS. *Am J Hosp Care* **3**, 35–7.

Martin, J.P. (1988) Hospice and home care for persons with AIDS/ARC: meeting the challenges and ensuring quality. *Death Stud* **12**, 463–80.

Martin, J.P. (1991) Issues in the current treatment of hospice patients with HIV disease. *Hosp J* 7, 31–40.

Martinson, I.M. (1980) Dying children at home. *Nurs Times* 76, 129–32.

Martinson, I.M., Moldow, D.G., Armstrong, G.D., Henry, W.F., Nesbit, M.E., and Kersey, J.H. (1986) Home care for children dying of cancer. *Res Nurs Health* 9, 11–16.

Masterson Allen, S., Mor, V., and Laliberte, L. (1987) Turnover in national hospice study sites: a reflection of organizational growth. *Hosp J* 3, 147–64.

Maull, F.W. (1991) Hospice care for prisoners: establishing an inmate-staffed hospice program in a prison medical facility. *Hosp J* 7, 43–55.

McCabe, S.V. (1982) An overview of hospice care. *Cancer Nurs* 5, 103–8.

McCaffrey-Boyle, D. (1994) New identities: The changing profile of patients with cancer, their families and their professional care givers. *Oncol Nurs Forum* 21, 55–61.

McCaffrey-Boyle, D. (1995) Documentation and outcomes of advanced nursing practise. *Oncol Nurs Forum* 22, 11–17.

McCallum, L.W., Dykes, J.N., Painter, L., and Gold, J. (1989) The Ankali project: A model for the use of volunteers to provide emotional support in terminal illness. *Med J Aust* 151, 33–8.

McCann, K. (1991) The work of a specialist AIDS home support team: the views and experiences of patients using the service. *J Adv Nurs* 16, 832–6.

McCann, K. and Wadsworth, E. (1992) The role of informal carers in supporting gay men who have HIV related illness: What do they do and what are their needs? *AIDS Care* 4, 25–34.

McCann, K., Wadsworth, E., and Beck, E.J. (1993) Planning health care for people with HIV infection and AIDS. *Health Serv Manage Res* 6, 167–77.

McCarthy, M. (1990) Hospice patients: a pilot study in twelve centres. *Palliat Med* 4, 93–104.

McCarthy, M., Addington-Hall, J.M., and Altmann, D. (1997a) The experience of dying with dementia: A retrospective study. *Int J of Geriatric Psychiatry* 12, 404–9.

McCarthy, M., Addington-Hall, J.M., and Lay, M. (1997b) Communication and choice in dying from heart disease. *J R Soc Med* 90, 128–31.

McCarthy, M., Howard, M., and Conway, J. (1988) Evaluation of terminal care: an exploratory study. *Med Sociol News* 13, 12–15.

McCarthy, M., Lay, M., and Addington-Hall, J.M. (1996) Dying from heart disease: symptoms and hospital care in the last year of life reported by informal carers. *J R Coll Physicians* 30, 325–8.

McClement, S.E. and Degner, L.F. (1995) Expert nursing behaviors in care of the dying adult in the intensive care unit. *Heart Lung: J Crit Care* 24, 408–19.

McCue, J.D. (1995) The naturalness of dying. *JAMA* 273, 1039–43.

McCusker, J. (1983) Where cancer patients die: An epidemiologic study. *Public Health Rep* **98**, 170–6.

McCusker, J. (1984) The terminal period of cancer: Definition and descriptive epidemiology. *J Chron Dis* **37**, 377–85.

McCusker, J. (1985) The use of home care in terminal cancer. *Am J Prev Med* **1**, 42–52.

McCusker, J. and Stoddard, A.M. (1987) Effects of an expanding home care program for the terminally ill. *Med Care* **25**, 373–85.

McCusker, J., Stoddard, A.M., and Sorensen, A.A. (1988) Do HMOs reduce hospitalization of terminal cancer patients? *Inquiry* **25**, 263–70.

McDonnell, M.M. (1989) Patient's perceptions of their care at Our Lady's Hospice, Dublin. *Palliat Med* **3**, 47–53.

McEnroe, L.E. (1996) Role of the oncology nurse in home care: family-centered practice. *Semin Oncol Nurs* **12**, 188–92.

McGee, R.F., Powell, M.L., Broadwell, D.C., and Clark, J.E. (1987) A Delphi survey of oncology clinical specialist competencies. *Oncol Nurs Forum* **14**, 29–34.

McGinnis, S. (1986) How can nurses improve the quality of life of the hospice client and family? *Hosp J* **2**, 23–36.

McGuire, D.B., Walczak, J.R., and Krumm, S.L. (1994) Development of a nursing research utilization program in a clinical oncology setting: organization, implementation, and evaluation. *Oncol Nurs Forum* **21**, 704–10.

McKee, C.M., Rajaratnam, G., and Lessof, L. (1988) Attitudes to a hospital based terminal care scheme. *Postgrad Med J* **64**, 678–80.

McKeogh, M. (1995) Dementia in HIV disease—a challenge for palliative care? *J Palliat Care* **11**, 30–3.

McMillan, S.C. (1996) The quality of life of patients with cancer receiving hospice care. *Oncol Nurs Forum* **23**, 1221–8.

McMillan, S.C. and Mahon, M. (1994a) A study of quality of life of hospice patients on admission and at week 3. *Cancer Nurs* **17**, 52–60.

McMillan, S.C. and Mahon, M. (1994b) Measuring quality of life in hospice patients using a newly developed Hospice Quality of Life Index. *Qual Life Res* **3**, 437–47.

McMillan, S.C., Heusinkveld, K.B., and Spray, J. (1995) Advanced practice in oncology nursing: a role delineation study. *Oncol Nurs Forum* **22**, 41–50.

McNally, J.C., Bohnet, N., and Lindquist, M.E. (1996) Hospice nursing. *Semin Oncol Nurs* **12**, 238–43.

McQuay, H. and Moore, A. (1994) Need for rigorous assessment of palliative care. *BMJ* **309**, 1315–16.

McQuillan, R., Finlay, I., Roberts, D., Branch, C., Forbes, K., and Spencer, M.G. (1996) The provision of a palliative care service in a teaching hospital and subsequent evaluation of that service. *Palliat Med* **10**, 231–9.

McWhan, K. (1991) Caring for dying patients in acute hospital wards: a review. *Nurs Pract* **5**, 25–8.

McWhinney, I.R., Bass, M.J., and Donner, A. (1994) Evaluation of a palliative care service: problems and pitfalls. *BMJ* **309**, 1340–2.

McWhinney, I.R., Bass, M.J., and Orr, V. (1995) Factors associated with location of death (home or hospital) of patients referred to a palliative care team. *Can Med Assoc J* **152**, 361–7.

McWilliam, C.L., Burdock, J., and Wamsley, J. (1993) The challenging experience of palliative care support-team nursing. *Oncol Nurs Forum* **20**, 779–85.

Meier, M.L. and Neuenschwander, H. (1995) Hospice—a homecare service for terminally ill cancer patients in southern Switzerland. *Support Care Cancer* **3**, 389–92.

Mercadante, S. and Mangione, S. (1990) Home palliative care: the challenge in Palermo. *J Palliat Care* **6**, 56–8.

Mercadante, S., Genovese, G., Kargar, J.A., Maddaloni, S., Roccella, S., Salvaggio, L., and Simonetti, M.T. (1992) Home palliative care: results in 1991 versus 1988. *J Pain Symptom Manage* **7**, 414–18.

Merrouche, Y., Freyer, G., Saltel, P., and Rebattu, P. (1996) Quality of final care for terminal cancer patients in a comprehensive cancer centre from the point of view of patients' families. *Support Care Cancer* **4**, 163–8.

Messenger, T. and Roberts, K.T. (1994) The terminally ill: serenity nursing interventions for hospice clients. *J Gerontol Nurs* **20**, 17–22.

Meystre, C., Gaskill, J., and Rudd, N. (1996) Hospital-based palliative care teams—are doctors and pain control teams adequate? Coventry: Palliative Care Research Forum.

Miaskowski, C., Lamkin, L., Buchsel, P.C., Campbell, L., Moskowitz, R., and Summers, B. (1993) Nursing salaries and practice patterns: a nationwide evaluation by the Oncology Nursing Society. *Cancer Invest* **11**, 689–98.

Michard, P., Marin, I., Camberlein, Y., and Abiven, M. (1990) Soins palliatifs des malades en phase terminale. Expérience de l'Unité de Soins Palliatifs de l'Hôpital International de l'Université de Paris. [Palliative treatment of patients in terminal phase. Experience at the Unité de Soins Palliatifs of the Hôpital International de l'Université de Paris] *Ann Med Intern* **141**, 313–18.

Miller, R.D. and Walsh, T.D. (1991) Psychosocial aspects of palliative care in advanced cancer. *J Pain Symptom Manage* **6**, 24–9.

Mills, M., Davies, H.T.O., and Macrae, W.A. (1994) Care of dying patients in hospital. *BMJ* **309**, 583–6.

Miner, P.D. and Canobbio, M.M. (1994) Care of the adult with cyanotic congenital heart disease. *Nurs Clin North Am* **29**, 249–67.

Mitchell, A., Hunter, D., Blackhurst, D., Stroud, C., and Lee, B. (1994) Hospice care: The cheaper alternative (5). *JAMA* **271**, 1576–7.

Moinpour, C.M. and Polissar, L. (1989) Factors affecting place of death of hospice and non-hospice cancer patients. *Am J Public Health* **79**, 1549–51.

Moldow, D.G., Armstrong, G.D., Henry, W.F., and Martinson, I.M. (1982) The cost of home care for dying children. *Med Care* **20**, 1154–60.

Mooney, K.H., Ferrell, B.R., Nail, L.M., Benedict, S.C., and Haberman, M.R. (1991) 1991 Oncology Nursing Society Research Priorities Survey. *Oncol Nurs Forum* **18**, 1381–8.

Moons, M., Kerkstra, A., and Biewenga, T. (1994) Specialized home care for patients with AIDS: an experiment in Rotterdam, The Netherlands. *J Adv Nurs* **19**, 1132–40.

Moore, M.K. (1993) Dying at home: A way of maintaining control for the person with ALS/MND. *Palliat Med* **7**, 65–8.

Mor, V. and Hiris, J. (1983) Determinants of site of death among hospice cancer patients. *J Health Soc Behav* **24**, 375–85.

Mor, V. and Kidder, D. (1985) Cost savings in hospice: final results of the National Hospice Study. *Health Serv Res* **20**, 407–22.

Mor, V. and Laliberte, L. (1983) Roles ascribed to volunteers. An examination of different types of hospice organization. *Eval Health Prof* **6**, 453–64.

Mor, V. and Masterson-Allen, S. (1987) *Hospice care systems: Structure, process, costs and outcome*. New York: Springer.

Mor, V. and Masterson-Allen, S. (1990) A comparison of hospice vs conventional care of the terminally ill cancer patient. *Oncology Huntingt* **4**, 85–91.

Mor, V., Wachtel, T.J. and Kidder, D. (1985) Patient predictors of hospice choice. Hospital versus home care programs. *Med Care* **23**, 1115–19.

Mor, V., Greer, D.S. and Kastenbaum, R. (1988a) *The hospice experiment*, Baltimore: The John Hopkins Press.

Mor, V., Stalker, M.Z., Gralla, R., Scher, H.I., Cimma, C., Park, D. *et al.* (1988b) Day hospital as an alternative to inpatient care for cancer patients: a random assignment trial. *J Clin Epidemiol* **41**, 771–85.

Morris, J.N. and Sherwood, S. (1987) Quality of life of cancer patients at different stages of the disease trajectory. *J Chron Dis* **40**, 545–53.

Morris, J.N., Mor, V., Goldberg, R.J. *et al.* (1986a) The effect of treatment setting and patient characteristics on pain in terminal cancer patients: A report from the National Hospice Study. *J Chron Dis* **39**, 27–35.

Morris, J.N., Suissa, S., Sherwood, S. *et al.* (1986b) Last days: A study of the quality of life of terminally ill cancer patients. *J Chron Dis* **39**, 47–56.

Morris, W.A. (1981) Care of the terminally ill in a district general hospital. *BMJ* **282**, 287–8.

Morrison, C. (1990) Case management and the determination of appropriate care settings for persons living with AIDS. In Heussner, R. and Hoffman, W. (eds) *Community based care of persons with AIDS*, pp. 75–82. Minneapolis: DHSS.

Mortenson, L.E., Dunlop, B., Enck, R.E., and Rogers, B. (1983) Descriptive evaluation of matched hospice and non-hospice patients. *Prog Clin Biol Res* 120, 417–27.

Moss, V. (1989) Mildmay Mission Hospital: Continuing care for people with AIDS. In Bould, M. and Peacock, G. (eds) *AIDS models of care*. London: King's Fund.

Moss, V. (1991) Patient characteristics presentation and problems encountered in advanced AIDS ina hospice setting. *Palliat Med* 5, 112–16.

Moss, V. (1994) Care for patients with advanced HIV and AIDS disease. *Palliat Care Term Illness* 2, 84–93.

Mount, B.M. (1980) A terminal care service in a general hospital. In Twycross, R.G. and Ventafridda, V. (eds) *The continuing care of terminal cancer patients*. New York: Pergamon Press.

Mount, B.M. and Scott, J.F. (1983) Whither hospice evaluation. *J Chron Dis* 36, 731–6.

Muurinen, J.M. (1986) The economics of informal care. Labor market effects in the National Hospice Study. *Med Care* 24, 1007–17.

Muzzin, L.J., Anderson, N.J., Figueredo, A.T., and Gudelis, S.O. (1994) The experience of cancer. *Soc Sci Med* 38, 1201–8.

Myers, K.G. and Trotman, I.F. (1995) Palliative care needs in a district general hospital: a survey of patients with cancer. *Eur J Cancer Care* 5, 116–21.

Nash, A. (1993) Reasons for referral to a palliative nursing team. *J Adv Nurs* 18, 707–13.

National Council for Hospice and Specialist Palliative Care Services. (1994) Care in the community for people who are terminally ill. *Guidelines for health authorities and social services departments*, pp. 1–4. London: National Council for Hospice and Specialist Palliative Care Services.

Neale, B. and Clark, D. (1992) Informal palliative care: a review of research on needs and services. *J Cancer Care* 1, 193–8.

Neale, B., Clark, D., and Heather, P. (1993) *Purchasing palliative care. A review of the policy and research literature*. Sheffield: Trent Palliative Care Centre.

NHS Centre for Reviews and Dissemination, University of York (1996) Understanding systematic reviews of research of effectiveness. CRD report 4. York.

Nicholas, E. and Frankenburg, R. (1992) Towards a strategy for palliative care. *Soc Sci Med* 40, 1193–202.

Noble, W.T. (1996) Psychological distress and symptom control in patients with advanced cancer: the effect of some simple interventions. MD thesis, Department of General Practice, University of Sheffield.

Norris, F.H. (1992) Motor neurone disease. Treating the untreated. *BMJ* **304**, 459–60.

Norris, F.H., Smith, R.A., and Denys, E.H. (1985) Motor neurone disease: towards better care. *BMJ* **291**, 259–62.

Norwood, M. (1990) Home care of the terminally ill. *Am J Hosp Pharm* **47**, S23–6.

Noyes, R. and Travis, T.A. (1973) The care of terminally ill patients. *Arch Intern med* **132**, 607–11.

Noyes, R., Travis, A., and Brightwell, D.R. (1993) The care of terminal patients: a statewide survey. *J Iowa Med Soc* **LXXIII**, 527–30.

O'Brien, T., Kelly, M., and Saunders, C. (1992) Motor neurone disease: a hospice perspective. *BMJ* **304**, 471–3.

O'Donnell, N.M. (1992) A regional approach to palliative care services. *J Palliat Care* **8**, 43–6.

O'Neill, W., O'Connor, P., and Latimer, E. (1992) Hospital palliative care services: three models in three countries. *J Pain Symptom Manage* **7**, 406–13.

Obbens, E. (1997) Neurological problems in palliative care. In Doyle D., Hanks G.W.C., and Macdonald N. (eds). *Oxford textbook of palliative medicine*. Oxford: Oxford University Press.

Oji McNair, K. (1985) A cost analysis of hospice versus non-hospice care: positioning characteristics for marketing a hospice. *Health Marketing Quarterly* **2**, 119–29.

Oliver, D. (1996) The quality of care and symptom control—the effects on the terminal phase of als/mnd. *J Neurol Sciences* **139**, 134–6.

Olsen, E.J. and Wilson, D.W. (1982) Hospice: within the VA hospital system. *Fam Community Health* **5**, 21–9.

Ophof, J., Leucht, R., Frohmuller, S., Dorsam, J., Ruoff, G., and Schlag, P. (1989) Experiences in home care of cancer-patients—a new approach in cancer nursing. *Acta Oncol* **1**, 35–8.

Oreopoulos, D.G. (1995) Commentary. Withdrawal from dialysis: when letting die is better than helping live. *Lancet* **346**, 3–4.

Owen, G., Crouch, P., and Wadey, A. (1989) *Marie Curie cancer care. A study of the Marie Curie community nursing service*. London: Marie Curie Memorial Foundation.

Pannuti, F. and Tanneberger, S. (1992) The Bologna Eubiosia Project: hospital-at-home care for advanced cancer patients. *J Palliat Care* **8**, 11–17.

Paradis, L.F. and Cummings, S.B. (1986) The evolution of hospice in America toward organizational homogeneity. *J Health Soc Behav* **27**, 370–86.

Parkes, C.M. (1978) Home or hospital? Terminal care as seen by surviving spouses. *J R Coll Gen Pract* **28**, 19–30.

Parkes, C.M. (1979) Terminal care evaluation of in-patient service at St Christopher's Hospice: Part 1 and 2. *Postgrad Med J* **55**, 517–25.

Parkes, C.M. (1980) Terminal care: evaluation of an advisory domiciliary service at St Christopher's Hospice. *Postgrad Med J* **56**, 685–9.

Parkes, C.M. (1985) Terminal care: home, hospital, or hospice? *Lancet* **1**, 155–7.

Parkes, C.M. and Parkes, J. (1984) 'Hospice' versus 'hospital' care—re-evaluation after 10 years as seen by surviving spouses. *Postgrad Med J* **60**, 120–4.

Partridge, N. (1989) The Terrence Higgins Trust. In Bould, M. and Peacock, G. (eds) *AIDS models of care*. London: King's Fund.

Patton, M.D. (1993) Action research and the process of continual quality improvement in a cancer center. *Oncol Nurs Forum* **20**, 751–5.

Patton, M. and Mooney, D. (1990) The nature of care delivered to terminally ill cancer-patients in the acute care hospital. *Progress in Clinical & Biological Research* **339**, 455–63.

Pawling Kaplan, M. and O'Connor, P. (1989) Hospice care for minorities: an analysis of a hospital-based inner city palliative care service. *Am J Hosp Care* **6**, 13–21.

Payne, R. and Gonzales, G. (1997) Pathophysiology of pain in cancer and other terminal diseases. In Doyle, D., Hanks, G.W.C., and Macdonald, N. (eds). *Oxford textbook of palliative medicine*. Oxford: Oxford University Press.

Payne, S. and Relf, M. (1994) The assessment of need for bereavement follow-up in palliative and hospice care. *Palliat Med* **8**, 291–7.

Peace, G., O'Keefe, C., Faulkner, A. and Clark, J. (1992) Childhood cancer: psychosocial needs: Are they being met? *J Cancer Care* **1**, 3–13.

Pepler, C.J. and Lynch, A. (1991) Relational messages of control in nurse-patient interactions with terminally ill patients with AIDS and cancer. *J Palliat Care* **7**, 18–29.

Peruselli, C., Camporesi, E., Colombo, A.M., Cucci, M., Sironi, P.G., Bellodi, M., Cirillo, R., Love, E., and Mariano, R. (1992) Nursing care planning for terminally ill cancer patients receiving home care. *J Palliat Care* **8**, 4–7.

Petersen, S. (1992) Beyond hospice care: a survey of community outreach programs. *Am J Hosp Palliat Care* **9**, 15–22.

Petrosino, B.M. (1985) Characteristics of hospice patients, primary caregivers and nursing care problems. *Hosp J* **1**, 3–19.

Petrosino, B.M. (1988) Nursing research in hospice care. *Hosp J* **4**, 29–45.

Pettingale, K.W. (1986) Progress in terminal care. *Practitioner* **230**, 891–5.

Pfeiffer, E. (1995) Institutional placement for patients with Alzheimer's disease. How to help families with a difficult decision. *Postgrad Med* 97, 125–6, 129–32.

Pichlmaier, H. (1994) Terminal care in-hospital and ambulatory care. *Fortschritt und Fortbildung in der Medizin [Advances And Continuing Education In Medicine]* 18, 13–14.

Pinkerton, C.R. (1993) Multidisciplinary care in the management of childhood cancer. *Br J Hosp Med* 50, 54–9.

Pizzi, M. (1983) Hospice and the terminally ill geriatric patient. *Physical and Occupational Therapy in Geriatrics* 3, 45–54.

Plumb, J.D. and Ogle, K.S. (1992) Hospice care. *Prim Care* 19, 807–20.

Pollack, E.S. (1984) The epidemiology of cancer and the delivery of medical-care services. *Public Health Rep* 5, 476–83.

Powel, L.L. and Mayer, D.K. (1992) The future of advanced clinical practice in oncology nursing. *Oncol Nurs Forum* 19, 28–31.

Powers, J.S. and Burger, M.C. (1987) Terminal care preferences: Hospice placement and severity of disease. *Public Health Rep* 102, 444–9.

Prigerson, H.G. (1991) Determinants of hospice utilization among terminally ill geriatric patients. *Home Health Care Serv Q* 12, 81–112.

Qvarnstrom, U. (1987) Hospice care in a university hospital—a three-stage model. *NLN Publ* 79–85.

Raftery, J.P., Addington Hall, J.M., MacDonald, L.D., Anderson, H.R., Bland, J.M., Chamberlain, J., and Freeling, P. (1996) A randomized controlled trial of the cost-effectiveness of a district co-ordinating service for terminally ill cancer patients. *Palliat Med* 10, 151–61.

Rango, N. (1985) The nursing home resident with dementia. Clinical care, ethics, and policy implications. *Ann Intern Med* 102, 835–41.

Raudonis, B.M. (1993) The meaning and impact of empathic relationships in hospice nursing. *Cancer Nurs* 16, 304–9.

Rayson, F., Brooks, D., Clark, D., Whynes, D., and Ahmedzai, S. (1995) Multi-disciplinary evaluation of a new hospice-at-home service. *Palliat Med* 9, 63–64.

Redman, S., White, K., Ryan, E., and Hennrikus, D. (1995) Professional needs of palliative care nurses in New South Wales. *Palliat Med* 9, 36–44.

Rees, G.J. (1985) Cost-effectiveness in oncology. *Lancet* 2, 1405–8.

Regnard, C. and Parker, R. (1994) Access to specialist palliative care. May be expanding too quickly (18). *BMJ* 308, 655–6.

Reilly, P.M. and Patten, M.P. (1981) Terminal care in the home. *J R Coll Gen Pract* 31, 531–7.

Reimer, J.C., Davies, B., and Martens, N. (1991) Palliative care. The nurse's role in helping families through the transition of 'fading away'. *Cancer Nurs* 14, 321–7.

Reisetter, K.H. and Thomas, B. (1986) Nursing care of the dying: its relationship to selected nurse characteristics. *Int J Nurs Stud* **23**, 39–50.

Reuben, D.B., Mor, V., and Hiris, J. (1988) Clinical symptoms and length of survival in patients with terminal cancer. *Arch Intern med* **148**, 1586–91.

Richardson, S., Leggieri, J. and Somers, C. (1987) A support program for the hospitalized terminally ill. Extensive volunteered staff time is key. *Am J Hosp Care* **4**, 20–4.

Riley, G., Lubitz, J., Prihoda, R., and Rabey, E. (1987) The use and costs of Medicare services by cause of death. *Inquiry* **24**, 233–44.

Rinck, G., Kleijnen, J., Van den Bos, T.G., de Haes, H.J., Schade, E., and Veenhof, C.H. (1995) Trials in palliative care. *BMJ* **310**, 598–9.

Robbins, M., Lee, T. and Wallis, H. (1997) *The Bristol nursing at home service: An evaluation of the first year.* Bath: University of Bath.

Robbins, M.A. and Frankel, S.J. (1995) Palliative care services: what needs assessment? *Palliat Med* **9**, 287–93.

Robinson, B.E. and Pham, H. (1996) Cost-effectiveness of hospice care. *Clin Geriatr Med* **12**, 417–28.

Robinson, L. and Stacy, R. (1994) Palliative care in the community: setting practice guidelines for primary care teams. *Br J Gen Pract* **44**, 461–4.

Roder, D., Bonett, A., Hunt, R., and Beare, M. (1987) Where patients with cancer die in South Australia. *Med J Aust* **147**, 11–13.

Rogatz, P. (1985) Home health care: some social and economic considerations. *Home Healthc Nurse* **3**, 38–43.

Rogatz, P., Schwartz, F., and Dennis, J. (1991) A community-based hospice program. *NY State J Med* **91**, 500–2.

Rogers, M. (1996) *Palliative care audit in primary care report: Anglia Clinical Audit and Effectiveness Team.* Cambridge: Institute of Public Health.

Rogers, W.F., Clarke, C., and Whitfield, A.G.W. (1981) Hospice planning in North Staffordshire. *J R Coll Physicians Lond* **15**, 25–7.

Rosenberg, E. and Short, C. (1983) Issues of institutionalization: Five percent fallacies and terminal care. *Int J Aging Hum Dev* **17**, 43–55.

Rosenthal, M.A., Gebski, V.J., Kefford, R.F., and Stuart Harris, R.C. (1993) Prediction of life-expectancy in hospice patients: identification of novel prognostic factors. *Palliat Med* **7**, 199–204.

Rousseau, P. (1994) Hospice care (3). *JAMA* **272**, 767.

Ryan, P.Y. (1992) Perceptions of the most helpful nursing behaviors in a home-care hospice setting: caregivers and nurses. *Am J Hosp Palliat Care* **9**, 22–31.

Ryndes, T. (1995) New beginnings in hospice. *Health Forum J* **38**, 27–9.

Sachs, G.A. (1995) The care of dying patients: A position statement from the American Geriatrics Society. *J Am Geriatr Soc* **43**, 577–8.

Sager, M.A., Easterling, D.V., and Leventhal, E.A. (1988) An evaluation of increased mortality rates in Wisconsin nursing homes. *J Am Geriatr Soc* **36**, 739–46.

Sager, M.A., Easterling, D.V., Kindig, D.A., and Anderson, O.W. (1989) Changes in the location of death after passage of Medicare's prospective payment system. A national study. *N Engl J Med* **320**, 433–9.

Samarel, N. (1989) Nursing in a hospital-based hospice unit. *Image J Nurs Sch* **21**, 132–6.

Samuelsson, G. and Sundstrom, G. (1988) Ending one's life in a nursing home: a note on Swedish findings. *Int J Aging Hum Dev* **27**, 81–8.

Sanderson, H., Mountney, L., and Harris, J. (1992) *Epidemiologically based needs assessment, DHA project, Cancer of the lung* (provisional version). Leeds: NHS Management Executive.

Sands, D.A., Galassi, A., Chisholm, L., Dimond, E., Caubo, K., and Jenkins, J. (1993) A cancer day hospital: an alternative approach to caring for patients in clinical trials. *Oncol Nurs Forum* **20**, 787–93.

Saunders, C., Walsh, T.D., and Smith, M. (1981) Hospice care in motor neurone disease. In Saunders, C. and Summers, D.H. (eds) *Hospice: the living idea*, pp. 126–47. London: Edward Arnold.

Saunders, J.M. and McCorkle, R. (1985) Models of care for persons with progressive cancer. *Nurs Clin North Am* **20**, 365–77.

Schaerer, R., Desforges, E., and Laval, G. (1991) Comment evaluer les couts des soins palliatifs? [How to estimate palliative care costs?] *Journal d'Economie Medicale* **9**, 407–18.

Schapira, D.V., Studnicki, J., Bradham, D.D., Wolff, P., and Jarrett, A. (1993) Intensive care, survival, and expense of treating critically ill cancer patients. *JAMA* **269**, 783–6.

Schietinger, H. (1986) AIDS beyond the hospital: I A home care plan for AIDS. *Am J Nurs* **86**, 1021–8.

Schofferman, J. (1987) Hospice care of the patient with AIDS. *Hosp J* **3**, 51–74.

Schweitzer, S.O., Mitchell, B., Landsverk, J., and Laparan, L. (1993) The costs of a pediatric hospice program. *Public Health Rep* **108**, 37–44.

Scitovsky, A.A. (1984) 'The high cost of dying': what do the data show? *Milbank Mem Fund Q Health Soc* **62**, 591–608.

Scitovsky, A.A. (1989) Medical care in the last twelve months of life: The relation between age, functional status, and medical care expenditures. *Milbank Q* **66**, 640–60.

Scitovsky, A.A. (1994) 'The high cost of dying' revisited. *Milbank Q* **72**, 561–91.

Scott, S.N. (1995) Report of the task force on care of the dying and the bereaved in Argyll and Clyde Health Board. Paisley: Argyll and Clyde Health Board.

Seale, C.F. (1989) What happens in hospices: a review of research evidence. *Soc Sci Med* **28**, 551–9.

Seale, C. (1991a) Communication and awareness about death: A study of a random sample of dying people. *Soc Sci Med* **32**, 943–52.

Seale, C. (1991b) A comparison of hospice and conventional care. *Soc Sci Med* **32**, 147–52.

Seale, C. (1991c) Death from cancer and death from other causes: relevance of the hospice approach. *Palliat Med* **5**, 12–19.

Seale, C. (1992) Community nurses and the care of the dying. *Soc Sci Med* **34**, 375–82.

Seale, C. (1994) *The year before death*. Aldershot: Avebury.

Seamark, D.A. (1998) Palliative terminal cancer care in community hospitals and a hospice: a comparative study. *Brit J Gen Pract* **48**, 1312–16.

Seamark, D.A, Williams, S., Hall, M., Lawrence, C.J., and Gilbert, J. (1998) Dying from cancer in community hospitals or a hospice: closest lay carer's perception. *Brit J Gen Pract* **48**, 1317–21.

Seamark, D.A., Thorne, C.P., Jones, R.V., Gray, D.J., and Searle, J.F. (1993) Knowledge and perceptions of a domiciliary hospice service among general practitioners and community nurses. *Br J Gen Pract* **43**, 57–9.

Seamark, D.A., Thorne, C.P., Lawrence, C., and Gray, D.J. (1995) Appropriate place of death for cancer patients: views of general practitioners and hospital doctors. *Br J Gen Pract* **45**, 359–63.

Seamark, D.A., Lawrence, C., and Gilbert, J. (1996) Characteristics of referrals to an inpatient hospice and a survey of general practitioner perceptions of palliative care. *J R Soc Med* **89**, 79–84.

Sebag Lanoe, R., Monier, C., Legrain, S., Maillos, A.M., and Dien, M.J. (1989) Soins palliatifs en geriatrie: etude retrospec sur 3 ans. [Palliative treatment in geriatrics: retrospective study spanning 3 years] *Rev Geriatr* **14**, 244–8.

Severs, M.P. and Wilkins, P.S.W. (1991) A hospital palliative care ward for elderly people. *Age Ageing* **20**, 361–4.

Shanahan, M.H. (1989). Soins infirmiers dans une unite de soins palliatifs. [Nursing in a unit for palliative cure] *Techniques Hospitalieres—Medico-Sociales et Sanitaires* **44**, 61–5.

Shapiro, E. (1983) Impending death and the use of hospitals by the elderly. *J Am Geriatr Soc* **31**, 348–51.

Shapiro, H.B. (1988) Financing the care of patients with the aquired immunodeficiency syndrome (AIDS). *Ann Intern Med* **108**, 470–3.

Shee, C.D. (1995) Palliation in chronic respiratory disease. *Palliat Med* **9**, 3–12.

Sheehan, C.J. and Rausch, P.G. (1984) Analysis of the Medicare/hospice program: rural applications. *Home Healthc Nurse* **2**, 38–40.

Siegel, K., Mesagno, F.P., Karus, D.G. and Christ, G. (1992) Reducing the prevalence of unmet needs for concrete services of patients with cancer. Evaluation of a computerized telephone outreach system. *Cancer* **69**, 1873–83.

Silver, S. (1981) Evaluation of a hospice program: Effects on terminally ill patients and their families. *Eval Health Prof* **4**, 306–15.

Simpson, K.S. (1991) The use of research to facilitate the creation of a hospital palliative care team. *Palliat Med* **5**, 122–9.

Sims, M.T. (1995) Can the hospices survive the market? A financial analysis of palliative care provision in Scotland. *J Manag Med* **9**, 4–16.

Singer, P.A. and Lowy, F.H. (1992) Rationing, Patient preferences and cost of care at the end of life. *Arch Intern med* **152**, 478–80.

Singh, S. (1989) Liaison with general practice. In Bould, M. and Peacock, G. (eds) *AIDS models of care*. London: King's Fund.

Singleton, R. (1992) Palliative home care program for terminally ill children. *Leadersh Health Serv* **1**, 21–7.

Slevin, M.L., Plant, H., Lynch, D., Drinkwater, J. and Gregory, W.M. (1988) Who should measure quality of life: the doctor or the patient? *Br J Cancer* **57**, 109–12.

Sloan, D. and Grant, M. (1989) Evaluating a Macmillan nursing service— the benefits of care. *Sr Nurse* **9**, 20–1.

SMAC (Standing Medical Advisory Committee and Standing Nursing and Midwifery Advisory Committee) (1992) *The principles and provisions of palliative care*. London: HMSO.

Smith, A.M., Eve, A., and Sykes, N.P. (1992) Palliative care services in Britain and Ireland 1990—an overview. *Palliat Med* **6**, 277–91.

Smith, J.E. and Waltman, N.L. (1994) Oncology clinical nurse specialists' perceptions of their influence on patient outcomes. *Oncol Nurs Forum* **21**, 887–93.

Smith, P. and Oliver, D. (1994) Palliative care 1994. *Service provision for black and ethnic groups; specific issues for consideration*. pp. 1–20. London: South West Thames Regional Health Authority.

Smith, S.N. and Bohnet, N. (1983) Organization and administration of hospice care. *J Nurs Admin* **13**, 10–16.

Smith, S.P. and Varoglu, G. (1985) Hospice: a supportive working environment for nurses. *J Palliat Care* **1**, 16–23.

Smith, W.R., Kellerman, A., and Brown, J.S. (1995) The impact of nursing home transfer policies at the end of life on a public acute care hospital. *J Am Geriatr Soc* **43**, 1052–7.

Smits, A., Mansfield, S., and Singh, S. (1990) Facilitating care of patients with HIV infection by hospital and primary care teams. *BMJ* **300**, 241–3.

Sontag, M.A. (1995) Characteristics of hospice programs, directors, and selected staff in one western state. *Am J Hosp Palliat Care* **12**, 29–37.

Sorbye, L.W. (1990) Homecare at the end of life. A study of fifteen patients. *Scand J Caring Sci* 4, 107–13.

Sowell, R.L. and Lowenstein, A. (1988) Comprehensive planning for AIDS related services. *J Nurs Admin* 18, 40–4.

Spiegel, D., Bloom, J.R., and Yalom, I. (1981) Group support for patients with metastatic cancer. A randomized outcome study. *Arch Gen Psychiatry* 38, 527–33.

Spiller, J.A. (1993) Domiciliary care: A comparison of the views of terminally ill patients and their family caregivers. *Palliat Med* 7, 109–15.

Spilling, R. (1986) Dying at home. In Spilling, R. (ed.) *Terminal care at home*, Oxford: Oxford University Press.

Stein, A. and Woolley, H. (1990) An evaluation of hospice care for children. In Anonymous *Listen my child has a lot of living to do. Caring for chidren with life-threatening conditions*, pp. 66–90. Oxford: Oxford University Press.

Stein, A., Forrest, G.C., Woolley, H., and Baum, J.D. (1989) Life threatening illness and hospice care. *Arch Dis Child* 64, 697–702.

Stephany, T.M. (1985a) Quality assurance for hospice programs. *Oncol Nurs Forum* 12, 33–40.

Stephany, T.M. (1985b) Utilization review in a hospice program. *J Community Health Nurs* 2, 13–20.

Stephany, T.M. (1992) AIDS does not fit the cancer model of hospice care. *Am J Hosp Palliat Care* 9, 13–14.

Stevensen, C. (1996) Assessing needs of people with cancer. *Contemp Nurse* 5, 36–9.

Stjernsward, J. (1988) WHO cancer pain relief programme. *Cancer Surv* 7, 195–208.

Stjernsward, J., Colleau, S.M., and Ventafridda, V. (1996) The World Health Organization Cancer Pain and Palliative Care Program. Past, present, and future. *J Pain Symptom Manage* 12, 65–72.

Stoddard, S. (1989) Hospice in the United States: an overview. *J Palliat Care* 5, 10–19.

Stoll, H.R. (1991) Effective pain control in cancer-patients in the home care setting. *Recent Results Cancer Res II* 36–42.

Stommel, M., Given, C.W., and Given, B.A. (1993) The cost of cancer home care to families. *Cancer* 71, 1867–74.

Strahan, G.W. (1994) An overview of home health and hospice care patients: preliminary data from the 1993 National Home and Hospice Care Survey. *Adv Data* 1–12.

Strahan, G.W. (1996) An overview of home health and hospice care patients: 1994 National Home and Hospice Care Survey. *Adv Data* 1–8.

Sulmasy, D.P. (1995) Managed care and managed death. *Arch Intern med* 155, 133–6.

Sun, Y. (1993) China: status of cancer pain and palliative care. *J Pain Symptom Manage* **8**, 399–403.

Sykes, N.P., Pearson, S.E., and Chell, S. (1992) Quality of care of the terminally ill: the carer's perspective. *Palliat Med* **6**, 227–36.

Talmi, Y.P., Roth, Y., Waller, A., *et al.* (1995) Care of the terminal head and neck cancer patient in the hospice setting. *Laryngoscope* **105** 315–18.

Tanneberger, S., Pannuti, F., Martoni, A., and Girodani, S. (1994) The cost-benefit relationship of care in advanced cancer—hospital or home management. *Proceedings of the Xvi International Cancer Congress— Free Papers And Posters* Tomes 1–4, 717–21.

Tarr, S., Roberts, D.E., Spencer, M.G., Tarr, M.J., and Finlay, I. (1992) Symptom control of cancer patients at a teaching hospital. *Pharmaceutical J Res Supp* **249**, R43.

Taylor, H. (1997) *The hospice movement in Britain—its role and its future.* London: Centre for Policy on Ageing.

Taylor, J. (1990) Coping with the stress on carers. *Practitioner* **234**, 300–1.

Tehan, C. (1991) The cost of caring for patients with HIV infection in hospice. *Hosp J* **7**, 41–59.

Thal, A.E. (1993) Health care for end-stage dementia (4). *J Am Geriatr Soc* **41**, 888.

Thaney, K.M. (1983) Nursing care for cancer-patients. *Manage Adv Cancer* **1983**, 299–310.

Thomson, C. (1989) London Lighthouse: a centre for people facing the challenge of AIDS. In Bould, M. and Peacock, G. (eds) *AIDS models of care.* London: King's Fund.

Thomson, W.A.R. (1981) The hospice tradition. *J R Soc Med* **74**, 90–1.

Thorne, C.P., Seamark, D.A., Lawrence, C., and Gray, D.J. (1994) The influence of general practitioner community hospitals on the place of death of cancer patients. *Palliat Med* **8**, 122–8.

Thorpe, G. (1993) Enabling more dying people to remain at home. *BMJ* **307**, 915–18.

Tierney, A.J., Sladden, S., Anderson, J., King, M., Lapsley, I., and Llewellyn, S. (1994) Measuring the costs and quality of palliative care: A discussion paper. *Palliat Med* **8**, 273–81.

Timothy, A.R., Brewin, T., Chamberlain, J., Horwich, A., Jennett, B., Kind, P. *et al.* (1988) Cost versus benefit in non-surgical management of patients with cancer. *BMJ* **297**, 471–2.

Torrens, P.R. (1985) Hospice care: what have we learned? *Annu Rev Public Health* **6**, 65–83.

Toscani, F. (1991) Inadequacies of care in far advanced cancer patients: a comparison between home and hospital in Italy. *Palliat Med* **5**, 31–6.

Townsend, J., Frank, A.O., Fermont, D., Dyer, S., Karran, O., Walgrove, A., and Piper, M. (1990) Terminal cancer care and patients' preference for place of death: a prospective study. *BMJ* **301**, 415–17.

Tramarin, A., Milocchi, F., Tolley, K., Vaglia, A., Marcolin, F., Manfrin, V., and de Lalla, F. (1992) An economic evaluation of home-care assistance for AIDS patients: a pilot study in a town in Northern Italy. *AIDS* **6**, 1377–83.

Tsamandouraki, K., Tountas, Y., and Trichopoulos, D. (1992) Relative survival of terminal cancer patients in home versus hospital care. *Scand J Soc Med* **20**, 51–4.

Turnbull, R. (1981) The Te Omanga hospice continuing care programme. *N Z Med J* **93**, 46–9.

Turner, J.A. (1992) Nursing care of the terminal lung cancer patient. *Nurs Clin North Am* **27**, 691–702.

Twycross, R. and Dunn, V. (1994) *Research in palliative care: the pursuit of reliable knowledge.* Occasional Paper 5, London: National Council for Hospice and Specialist Palliative Care Services.

van Weel, C. (1994) Teamwork. *Lancet* **344**, 1276–9.

Ventafridda, V., Tamburini, M., and Selmi, S. (1985) The importance of a home care program for patients with advanced cancer. *Tumori* **71**, 449–54.

Ventafridda, V., De Conno, F., Vigano, A., Ripamonti, C., Gallucci, M., and Gamba, A. (1989) Comparison of home and hospital care of advanced cancer patients. *Tumori* **75**, 619–625.

Ventafridda, V., De Conno, F., Ripamonti, C., Gamba, A., and Tamburini, M. (1990) Quality-of-life assessment during a palliative care programme. *Ann Oncol* **1**, 415–20.

Vinceguerra, V., Degnon, T., and Scidatino, A. (1986) A comparitive assessment of home versus hospital comprehensive treatment for advanced cancer patients. *J Clin Oncol* **4**, 21–8.

Viney, L.L., Walker, B.M., Robertson, T., Lilley, B., and Ewan, C. (1994) Dying in palliative care units and in hospital: a comparison of the quality of life of terminal cancer patients. *J Consult Clin Psychol* **62**, 157–64.

Volicer, L. (1986) Need for hospice approach to treatment of patients with advanced progressive dementia. *J Am Geriatr Soc* **34**, 655–8.

Volicer, L., Rheaume, Y., Brown, J., Fabiszewski, K., and Brady, R. (1986) Hospice approach to the treatment of patients with advanced dementia of the Alzheimer type. *JAMA* **256**, 2210–13.

Volicer, B.J., Hurley, A., Fabiszewski, K.J., Montgomery, P., and Volicer, L. (1993) Predicting short-term survival for patients with advanced Alzheimer's disease. *J Am Geriatr Soc* **41**, 535–40.

Volicer, L., Collard, A., Hurley, A., Bishop, C., Kern, D., and Karon, S. (1994) Impact of special care unit for patients with advanced Alzheimer's disease on patients' discomfort and costs. *J Am Geriatr Soc* **42**, 597–603.

Volicier, B.J., Hurley, A., and Fabiszewski, K.J. (1993) Predicting death within six months of fever. *J Am Geriatr Soc* **41**, 535–40.

Wachtel, T.J. and Mor, V. (1987) Physicians' use of health resources for terminal cancer patients: clinical setting versus physician specialty. *South Med J* **80**, 1120–4.

Wakefield, M.A., Beilby, J., and Ashby, M.A. (1993) General practitioners and palliative care. *Palliat Med* **7**, 117–26.

Wales, J., Kane, R., Robbins, S., Bernstein, L., and Krasnow, R. (1983) UCLA hospice evaluation study. Methodology and instrumentation. *Med Care* **21**, 734–44.

Wall, E., Rodriguez, G., and Saultz, J. (1993) A retrospective study of patient care needs on admission to an inpatient hospice facility. *J Am Board Fam Pract* **6**, 233–8.

Wallston, K.A., Burger, C., Smith, R.A., and Baugher, R.J. (1988) Comparing the quality of death for hospice and non-hospice cancer patients. *Med Care* **26**, 177–82.

Walsh, D., Gombeski, W.R., Jr., Goldstein, P., Hayes, D., and Armour, M. (1994) Managing a palliative oncology program: the role of a business plan. *J Pain Symptom Manage* **9**, 109–18.

Walsh, S. and Kingston, R.D. (1988) The use of hospital beds for terminally ill cancer patients. *Eur J Surg Oncol* **14**, 367–70.

Walsh, T.D. (1990) Continuing care in a medical center: the Cleveland Clinic Foundation Palliative Care Service. *J Pain Symptom Manage* **5**, 273–8.

Walsh, T.D. (1991) An overview of palliative care in cancer and AIDS. *Oncology Huntingt* **5**, 7–11.

Waltman, N.L. and Zimmermann, L. (1991) Variations among nurses in behavioural intentions towards the dying. *Hospice J* **7**, 37–49.

Walton, I. (1987) Terminal care of the elderly and bereavement counselling. *Practitioner* **231**, 869–73.

Ward, A. (1982) Standards for home care services for the terminally ill. *Community Med* **4**, 276–9.

Ward, A.W. (1987) Home care services—an alternative to hospices? *Community Med* **9**, 47–54.

Warson, S.R. (1985) The hospice model. *J Fla Med Assoc* **72**, 438–9.

Weeks, W.B., Kofoed, L.L., Wallace, A.E., and Welch, H.G. (1994) Advance directives and the cost of terminal hospitalization. *Arch Intern med* **154**, 2077–83.

Weissman, D.E. and Griffie, J. (1994) The Palliative Care Consultation Service of the Medical College of Wisconsin. *J Pain Symptom Manage* **9**, 474–9.

Welch, J.M. (1991) Symptoms of HIV disease. *Palliat Med* **5**, 46–51.

Weller, I. (1981) Hospice at home. *Nurs Mirror* **153**, 36–9.

Wells, R.J. (1987) Aspects of palliative care in AIDS. *Palliat Med* **1**, 49–52.

Welsh, J. (1993) A hospice in Glasgow, Scotland. *Gynaecol Cancer* 113–14.

Wershow, H.J. (1976) The four percent fallacy. Some further evidence and policy implications. *Gerontologist* 16, 52–5.

Weston-Smith, J., O'Donovan, J.B., Hoyle, G., Clegg, D.F., and Khalid, T. (1973) Comparative study of district and community hospitals. *BMJ* 2, 471–4.

Wiegert, O., Blues, A., and Wiegert, H.T. (1981) Community hospice programs: Factors to consider when planning to provide interfacing home and inpatient care options. *J Amb Care Manage* 4, 47–57.

Wiles, J. (1995) *Specialist palliative care: a statement of definitions.* Occasional Paper 8. London: National Council for Hospice and Specialist Palliative Care Services.

Wilhelm, M.E. and Wilhelm, M.A. (1984) Hospice development in a subacute care setting. *Hosp Prog* 65, 42–5, 74.

Wilkes, E. (1980) *Department of Health and Social Security. Report of the working group on terminal care.* London: HMSO.

Wilkes, E. (1984) Dying now. *Lancet* 1, 950–2.

Wilkes, E., Hinton, J., Higginson, I.J., Faulkner, A., Naysmith, A., Brodribb, C. *et al.* (1991) Palliative care: Guidelines for good practice and audit measures. *J R Coll Physicians Lond* 25, 325–8.

Wilkinson, H.J. (1986) Assessment of patient satisfaction and hospice: a review and an investigation. *Hosp J* 2, 69–94.

Wilkinson, S. (1991) Factors which influence how nurses communicate with cancer patients. *J Adv Nurs* 16, 677–88.

Wilson, B.P., Blosse, R.W., Tucker, J.L., and Spector, K.K. (1983) Hospice care: perspectives on a Blue Cross Plan's community pilot program. *Inquiry* 20, 322–7.

Wilson, D.C. (1982) The viablity of pediatric hospices: A case study. *Death Educ* 6, 205–12.

Wilson, I.M., Bunting, J.S., Curnow, R.N., and Knock, J. (1995) The need for inpatient palliative care facilities for noncancer patients in the Thames Valley. *Palliat Med* 9, 13–18.

Wilson, J.A., Lawson, P.M., and Smith, R.G. (1987) The treatment of terminally ill geriatric patients. *Palliat Med* 1, 149–53.

Wilson, S.A., Kovach, C.R., and Stearns, S.A. (1996) Hospice concepts in the care of end-stage dementia. *Geriatr Nurs* 17, 6–10.

Wilson-Barnett, J. (1988a) Key areas for terminal care nursing. In Wilson-Barnett, J. and Raiman, J. (eds) *Nursing issues and research in terminal care,* pp. 3–15. Chichester: Wiley.

Wilson-Barnett, J. (1988b) Progress in terminal care nursing. In Wilson-Barnett, J. and Raiman, J. (eds) *Nursing issues and research in terminal care,* pp. 203–214. Chichester: Wiley.

Winkel, P., Statland, B.E., Brammer, M.E., Christau, B., and Oster-gaard, E.R. (1990) Present and projected consumption of hospital bed-days as a function of terminal days before death. *Scand J Soc Med* 18, 39–44.

Winstead, K.D., Gilmore, M., Dollar, R., and Miller, E. (1980) Hospice consultation team: a new multi-disciplinary model. *Gen Hosp Psychiatry* 3, 169–76.

Woodruff, R. (1993) *Palliative medicine*. Melbourne: Asperula.

Woodruff, R.K., Jordan, L., Eicke, J.P., and Chan, A. (1991) Palliative care in a general teaching hospital: 2. Establishment of a service. *Med J Aust* 155, 662–5.

Woolley, H., Stein, A., Forrest, G.C., and Baum, J.D. (1989a) Imparting the diagnosis of life threatening illness in children. *BMJ* 298, 1623–6.

Woolley, H., Stein, A., Forrest, G.C., and Baum, J.D. (1989b) Staff stress and job satisfaction at a children's hospice. *Arch Dis Child* 64, 114–18.

Wright St Clair, R.E. (1983) Terminal care. *N Z Med J* 96, 49–50.

Zerwekh, J.V. (1995) A family caregiving model for hospice nursing. *Hosp J* 10, 27–44.

Zimmer, J.G., Groth Juncker, A., and McCusker, J. (1984) Effects of a physician-led home care team on terminal care. *J Am Geriatr Soc* 32, 288–92.

Zimmer, J.G., Groth Juncker, A., and McCusker, J. (1985) A randomized controlled study of a home health care team. *Am J Public Health* 75, 134–41.

Zorzitto, M.L., Knowles, S., and Fisher, R.H. (1989) The departmental approach to palliative care of hospitalized elderly: a comparative retrospective review over 15 years. *J Palliat Care* 5, 49–52.

Zylicz, Z. (1996) The Netherlands: status of cancer pain and palliative care. *J Pain Symptom Manage* 12, 136–8.

Index

Please note, the term palliative care is assumed: subject matter is directly referred to. Entries for tables and figures are set in italics.